Against the Grain

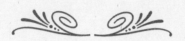

Jax Peters Lowell

Against the GRAIN

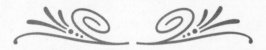

The Slightly Eccentric Guide to Living Well Without Gluten or Wheat

An Owl Book
Henry Holt and Company
New York

Henry Holt and Company, LLC
Publishers since 1866
115 West 18th Street
New York, New York 10011

Henry Holt® is a registered trademark
of Henry Holt and Company, LLC.

Library of Congress Cataloging-in-Publication Data
Lowell, Jacqueline Peters.
Against the grain: the slightly eccentric guide to living well
without gluten or wheat / Jax Peters Lowell—1st ed.
p.   cm.
ISBN 0-8050-3625-3 (An Owl Book: pbk.)
Includes bibliographical references and index.
1. Wheat-free diet.   2. Gluten-free diet.   I. Title.
RM237.87.L68   1995   94-39985
613.2′6—dc20   CIP

Henry Holt books are available for special promotions
and premiums. For details contact: Director, Special Markets.

First published in hardcover in 1995 by
Henry Holt and Company

First Owl Books Edition 1996

Designed by Francesca Belanger

Printed in the United States of America

10

For my father, John Peters,
whose gift is the fighting spirit
that informs and inspires
all that follows.

Contents

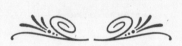

CHAPTER EIGHT

Etiquette for the Allergic 156

Eight simple rules to insure that you and your host never feel ill at ease

CHAPTER NINE

Your Cheating Heart and Other Special Problems 169

Sixteen anti-cheating strategies · Physical hunger · Emotional hunger · Daily cheat sheet · Dieting · How to give up smoking or other addictive behavior and still remain wheat- and gluten-free

CHAPTER TEN

Twelve Chefs Take the Challenge 186

Sheila Lukins's Cold Sauce "Hot Stuff" Pasta and Pasta Rustica · Molly O'Neill's Corn and Lobster Pie in a Chili-Polenta Crust · Alex Cormier's Banana Financier · Ed Barranco and George Georgiou's Mexican Lasagne · Beth Hillson's Pumpkin Prosciutto Gnocchi · John Rivera Sedlar's Abiquiu Hot Corn Soufflé · Jim Burns's Thai-jitas · Nick Malgieri's All-Corn Biscotti · Caroline Winge-Bogar's Grown-up Macaroni and Cheese · Angelo Peloni's Risotto Primavera · Lynn Jamison's Queen Mother Cake

CHAPTER ELEVEN

Growing up Wheat- and Gluten-free 212

Lots of don'ts for parents. Some dos · Cornmeal Porridge with Dried Fruit · Toll House Cookies Without the Toll · Jeremy's Peanut Butter and Jelly Cookies · Wheat-Free Brownies · Yeast-Rising Thick Pizza Crust · Mmmmmmmmmacaroni and Cheese · "Authentic" Happy Birthday Cake

CHAPTER TWELVE

The Wheat- and Gluten-free Resource Guide 229

National associations and support groups · Professional and lay associations · Government agencies · Diagnostic clinics · On-line computer services · Equipment · Drug companies · Food companies · Health food and specialty store foods · Mail-order foods not reviewed

Contents

Preface

Long Island, New York, Summer, 1993. The Bible says "bread eaten in secret is pleasant." For those of us who cannot tolerate wheat and other grains, bread eaten in secret is poison; the staff of life becomes life's big stiff. We know a moment's indiscretion can cause everything from hives, to headache, to diarrhea, to gastrointestinal scarring.

Most who suffer the discomforting symptoms of wheat allergy are forced to explore outsider grains, such as spelt and quinoa, not exactly in plentiful supply at the local supermarket, and to develop more than a passing interest in reviving the pre-Columbian cuisine in which they are featured. Others, like me, must endure the more serious and potentially cumulative effects of celiac disease, which basically narrows the universe to rice and corn and pushes the envelope of our resourcefulness at every meal.

Tell that to the hot dog vendor at Shea Stadium or to the fresh-faced kids at Briermier Farm, boxing still-warm fruit pies for the hordes heading to the Hamptons at any one of the dozens of farm stands along the way. Mention it to the well-meaning hostess who offers warm triangles of lightly browned pita with hummus to take the edge off, leaving you with sticky fingers and a howling hunger, or in any one of the quaint bed-and-breakfasts offering croissants, muffins, scones, all manner of homemade breads, and no substitutions for the price of your stay, or to the waiter in any one of the new restaurants that pop up every summer like fireflies on a hedge.

For those of us who must live without grain, that most comforting of comfort foods, now so in favor with those who seek to destroy all fat in their diets and who prescribe its fibrous crunch for everything from weight control, to healthy hearts, to whistle-clean colons, summer is not the easy-living, easy-eating time we hunger for all year. Like the never-ending flakiness of spring and the darkly satisfying crunch of autumn, summer is a minefield littered with crostini, pizza, biscotti, batter-fried chicken, cobblers, cookies, tarts, and tender loaves studded with bits of tomato and onion, swimming in a pool of heart-healthy, herb-scented extra-virgin olive oil.

Nothing prepared me for the deep sense of loss that accompanied my own diagnosis of celiac disease. It finally was recognized after years of discomforting and steadily worsening symptoms, including a particularly nasty form of diarrhea called steatorrhea, which left me with the kind of weight loss Weight Watchers wishes it could claim and skin with all the elasticity and supple appeal of an old handbag. Despite the knowledge that a gluten-free diet would soon restore my health and what was left of my figure, it took enormous willpower to watch someone butter a piece of toast. I wept at the sight of spaghetti, my all-time favorite prescription for mood elevation. I became morose at even the mention of butterscotch brownies and was struck by sudden urges to fondle warm rolls in restaurants. No longer could I join my friends in sending out for pizza with everything on it, even if *everything* meant a kinder, gentler version piled high with sun-dried tomatoes and chèvre.

How could I explain when friends were battling serious things such as breast cancer and brain injury and hearts that ticked like time bombs, while I had gotten off with a mere dietary restriction? I secretly grieved for all the foods I could never taste again and did what any self-respecting adult would. I cheated. Every chance I got.

I tucked pastries in kitchen drawers, carried croissants in my purse and nibbled at them on the street behind black Ray Bans. Positive that flying across time zones suspended the problem, I smuggled cupcakes in my carry-on luggage. I discovered that empty Christmas ornament boxes are the perfect size for stashing cookies for a solitary nibble, and in the middle of the night, I shaved the sides of a lemon pound cake, convincing myself that the thinner the slice, the safer the serving.

Who knows where this dangerous behavior may have led had I not discovered risotto with gorgonzola and porcini mushrooms, polenta with fresh basil and tomato sauce, Thai rice noodles in spicy peanut sauce, and fiery Indian pancakes made with pure lentil flour? One New Year's Eve, in a flash of inspiration inspired by greed, a glass of champagne, and a certain willingness to explore my potential for unusual social behavior, I slipped a tiny silver spoon out of my purse and headed for the caviar. From that moment on, I understood that real pleasure does not depend on toast points.

The epiphany came in my own kitchen after a careful inventory of my local organic food store where, among many unexpected treasures, I found a nutty and delicious, 100 percent brown rice pasta. Close inspection of the baking aisle yielded a wheat-free, gluten-free mix that enabled me to duplicate virtually any cake recipe and to arrive at a reasonable and safe version of the coveted lemon pound cake simply by substituting one cup of the mix for one cup of the wheat flour in the recipe. Subsequent trips revealed a cookie mix from the same company and more allergy-friendly foods.

At my house, Christmas comes every two or three months in the form of a carton packed with brown rice bread, hamburger and hot dog buns, and dense cocoa cookies, while another equally bulging parcel brings a brownie mix that can be easily doctored to replicate the intensely fudgey confections I so desperately missed.

The discovery of sponge cake, lady fingers, and old-fashioned, chocolate-covered leaf cookies from a bakery in Flushing, New York, brought tears to my eyes as well as an ounce or two to my hips. Lynn, the owner of Jamison's Restaurant in Philadelphia, whose silky Best of Philly corn muffins are custom made on my behalf with fresh peaches or strawberries or blueberries, or whatever fruit this talented chef deems worthy, will certainly be considered for a small bequest when my time comes. I buy them by the dozen and freeze them for those dark mornings when feelings of deprivation sneak up and threaten my equilibrium.

My confidence growing, I took the problem out of the privacy of my own kitchen and into the world of dinners, brunches, lunches, parties, holidays, vacations, and business trips. Friends fussed. Hostesses adjusted. Chefs rose to the culinary challenge, testing my rice pasta for the perfect moment of al dente. The UPS person and I became bosom buddies. The time for zigging while everyone else zagged had arrived.

I cannot deny that steamed mussels or garlicky escargot are not as sublime without a crusty bread with which to sop up the broth; a burger piled high with Jersey tomatoes, raw Vidalia onion, and a richly veined bleu is not as sinful without the bun; and a perfect rose-covered morning in Nantucket is not as sweet without the requisite blueberry muffin. But when you've learned to carry your own muffins, hand the waiter two slices of rice bread for the double cheeseburger or Eggs Benedict, toss a beautiful brown rice pasta with homemade pesto and grilled summer vegetables, followed by a fresh peach crumble, life begins to soften like the ripening season before you. What separates now challenges. The mouth waters with possibilities.

Suddenly you see half empty versus half full not as a meaningless cliché but as the difference between an empty plate and one that is deliciously full. I, for one, would rather be pleasantly stuffed than permanently stiffed.

I do not ordinarily write about food, leaving that subject to the experts, M. F. K. Fisher, Colette, Craig Claiborne, and Wolfgang Puck. I prefer fictional worlds in which culinary delights cause no harm to people who wouldn't dream of forgoing a crumb. However, I felt it was time to share my talent for invention with other grain intolerants like myself who are tired of explaining the problem to people who simply don't get it, who are bored with the whole idea of feeling like a victim or being perceived as a less-than-perfect person, who have maintained their culinary standards and who have absolutely no time to cry over toast, burned or otherwise.

Against the Grain is really about how I saved my own life and ate happily ever after. While it may be true that the oddball and slightly eccentric behavior that led to it is purely genetic, it's a skill anyone can learn easily. In fact, with a pinch of creativity, a dash of chutzpah, and a more than passing acquaintance with a UPS person, a fax machine, and a phone book full of 800 numbers, life can be very good again.

If viewed in the larger sense—and I sincerely hope you see it that way—the lessons contained herein will not only help you get the food you need, they will help you get the food you want, teach you to celebrate your uniqueness instead of hiding it, to see yourself as challenged, not sick, to take yes for an answer instead of no, and to learn to live in a state of abundance rather than in the narrow world of denial.

When you think about it, the crack is the most interesting place on the glass because it draws the light and illuminates the smooth perfection of the rest. Although it may be difficult and often painful to find it, I believe everything happens to us for a reason, so we can find our beauty in the flaws and perhaps even find our strengths in the way we handle them. I take comfort in the fact that I have been given a little less in life in order to find out how much more I can have when I use the gift of my natural resourcefulness for myself and for others.

My purpose in writing this book is to show that nothing is beyond the person who can rise above a problem involving something as important, as primal, and as basic to comfort as food. I believe that once you begin to develop and use your own creativity to its fullest, easily solving food problems you once thought insurmountable, and discover your own ability to eat as well as everyone else, you will find there is little you cannot overcome. You may even find yourself waking up one day and asking yourself, as I have: If I can do this, what else can I do?

Acknowledgments

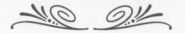

Writing a book like *Against the Grain* is a daunting task under the best of circumstances. Writing it in the gathering darkness of a family sorrow would have been impossible were it not for the open-hearted kindness of friends and the stunning generosity of strangers.

I will never sufficiently thank my husband, John Lowell, who phoned, faxed, copied, schlepped, comforted, cosseted, shored me up, and cheered me on, and this is as it should be. Nor will I ever be able to repay the debt I owe my mother, Catherine Peters, for her courage, her love, and her unselfishness.

For opening their hearts, as well as their kitchens and Filofaxes; for offering their shoulders, their friendship, their skill, and their love; and for renewing my faith in a family of our own choosing, I thank Tony von Fraunhofer, Nancy Barr, Jack and Barbara Cassidy, Marjorie Goldstein, Terese Zeccardi, and Barbara and Ray Brogliatti.

A special thanks to my agents, Sasha Goodman and David Andrew—the former for her unflagging enthusiasm and uncanny instinct for knowing how to help, which made all the difference, and the latter for his total professionalism and absolute faith in mine.

For their generosity beyond all reasonable expectations and for all the good work they do, my gratitude goes to Elaine Monarch, executive director of the Celiac Disease Foundation, and Phyllis Brogden, chair of the Greater Philadelphia Celiac Sprue Support Group.

For the great pains she took to share her skill, her short supply of time, and her determination that we all not only eat better but extraordinarily well, I thank Beth Hillson, president and founder of the Gluten-Free Pantry.

For absolute proof that acts of kindness are far less random than we think, I salute Dr. Gary Levine, Dr. Fergus Shanahan, Sheila Lukins, Jim and Barbara Burns, Bette Hagman, Alex Cormier, Ed Barranco, George Georgiou, Carrie Bogar, Lynn Jamison, Nick Malgieri, Angelo Peloni, John Sedlar, Evey Kane, Mollie O'Neill and the *New York Times*, Sarah Moulton, *Gourmet* magazine, Steven Rice, Jo Ann Ross Harvey, CSA/USA, the Gluten Intolerance Group of North America and the American Celiac Society, Tony and Lisa Tinnello, Leif Biderman, Betty Reynolds, Charles Weston, Raja Jhanjee, Wali Saai, Bon Siu, Bill Wong, and all those who dropped everything to help in the name of getting the word out that grain intolerance is no small matter for those of us who have it and that glue is not an ingredient in gluten for those of us who don't.

I thank all the good people whose resourcefulness, creativity, talent, and hard work have made living "against the grain" a delicious and educational experience for allergic and gluten-intolerant oddballs like me.

And finally, for her unruffled calm, I salute Beth Crossman, my editor.

Against the Grain

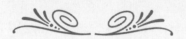

What Is Celiac Disease?

Gary M. Levine, M.D.

Asking a gastroenterologist to introduce a book on celiac disease and wheat allergy presents a rather demanding task. First, I am challenged to make a complicated subject understandable without being able to fall back on convenient medical terminology. Second, it is difficult to describe diseases with protean manifestations without causing all readers to believe they have the disease. Third, and perhaps the most difficult challenge of all, is to my ability to rise above the inevitable comparisons between this introduction's academic and scientific manners and the author's unusual, breezy, and often hilarious approach to the same subject.

Apologies aside, celiac disease, also known as gluten-sensitive enteropathy, celiac sprue, nontropical sprue, and idiopathic steatorrhea, is a disease whose extensive and variable symptoms challenge physicians to make a correct diagnosis in a timely fashion. The term "celiac sprue" has been applied to a clinical syndrome characterized by signs and symptoms of malabsorption, such as diarrhea and weight loss caused by eating grains. The term "gluten-sensitive enteropathy" more correctly defines the clinical pathologic disease caused by an immune-mediated sensitivity to gluten, a protein found in many cereal grains, principally wheat, barley, rye, and to a lesser degree oats. Most nutritionists agree that gluten is not present in rice, white or sweet potatoes, and corn.

Over one hundred years ago a British physician named Samuel Gee described the "coeliac affection." Dr. Gee observed the syndrome in people of all ages, but especially in children who had chronic diarrhea, weight loss, edema, and a distended abdomen. The disease invariably led to death unless cured by various diets. Many other physicians followed in the footsteps of this pioneer, prescribing diets based on rice, bananas, and lamb, which often led to symptomatic improvement of these children with celiac sprue.

It wasn't until the end of Word War II that the connection between the consumption of wheat and rye flour and the incidence of celiac sprue was made. Dutch pediatricians noted that during the war, when these flours were in short supply, celiac patients improved and few new cases were seen. After the war, when adequate food supplies were restored to the civilian population, celiac disease reappeared with regularity.

Based on this clinical observation, scientists then determined that a water-insoluble protein component of these grains, gluten, was the substance that damaged the intestine in certain individuals. Not until the 1950s were the characteristic microscopic changes in the lining of the intestine documented. The advent of invasive techniques to obtain biopsy specimens of the small intestine opened the floodgates of research activity, which taught us much of what we know today about this insidious disease.

Most recently, exciting research has been conducted that describes the immunologic mechanisms causing this type of intestinal injury. The vast majority of patients with celiac sprue possess a particular tissue type (to be exact, major histocompatibility antigens), which can be thought of in a similar fashion to each person's blood type. If one possesses the right, or more correctly, wrong tissue type, there is a high likelihood of developing celiac sprue.

The exact mechanism for this phenomenon is unknown, but several theories have been proposed. First, patients with celiac sprue may lack an enzyme necessary to digest toxic fractions of gluten. Second, celiac disease–associated tissue-type antigens are found on the surface of the intestinal cells that face the lumen (the part of the tubular intestine that is exposed to dietary contents). It is believed that these cells may bind with the toxic fractions of gluten. On the surface of the intestinal cell, gluten acts as a foreign substance, eliciting an immune reaction that destroys the intestinal-lining cells. Of course, each individual's tissue type is inherited. Because of this, if one of a pair of identical twins develops celiac disease, the other invariably will develop it as well.

Approximately 25 percent of Caucasians, in whom the disease is most common, possesses the celiac disease–associated tissue-type antigens, but obviously not all of them develop the disease. Other unknown factors begin the chain reaction of immunologic injury. One possible cause is infection with common agents such as viruses. At least one virus has been shown to possess a similar protein composition to toxic fractions of gluten. Theoretically, infection with this virus exposes the immune system to an antigen that is "shared" with the intestinal epithelium, or lining. Long after the virus has disappeared, the immune system continues to attack the body's own tissue, which produces celiac disease.

Once the immune system is activated in this way, there is progressive destruction of the surface cells that are normally responsible for absorption in the small intestine. Characteristically, the injury is most severe in the proximal intestine (jejunum) and becomes progressively less severe in the more distal intestine (ileum).

The reason for this pattern of distribution is probably due to the fact that gluten is gradually digested and eliminated from the intestinal lumen as the meal literally progresses downstream. The most proximal intestine, called the duodenum, is the primary site for absorption of minerals such as iron, calcium, and magnesium.

Extensive injury to the small bowel results in decreased absorption of nutrients such as carbohydrates, protein, and fat. When these substances are malabsorbed, they act as a laxative, holding water in the intestinal lumen and causing copious diarrhea. Diarrhea also occurs because the immunologic system releases mediators that lead the intestinal lumen to secrete fluid.

As a result of these processes, patients with full-blown celiac sprue have malabsorption of nutrients, minerals, and water. Large quantities of undigested nutrients in the intestine are available for metabolism by bacteria (you really don't want to know how many billions and billions of bacteria live in your gut!). The bacteria produce gases such as carbon dioxide, methane, and hydrogen, which account for the bloating and gurgling seen and heard in many patients.

Knowing these events it is not difficult to explain the many various manifestations of celiac sprue. However, most people don't have an easy time with or even access to medical textbooks. To complicate matters, many do not present with classic symptoms, which may vary from mild distention and gas after meals with normal bowel movements to incapacitating malnutrition, diarrhea, and dehydration. Occasionally patients present with signs and symptoms of vitamin and mineral deficiency, such as anemia due to iron, folate, and B_{12} malabsorption; bone pain and pathologic fractures because of malabsorption of calcium and vitamin D; and growth retardation in children. Some of the more subtle signs and symptoms of celiac sprue include bleeding tendencies, muscle spasms, nerve damage, infertility, impotence, and spontaneous abortion.

Although many individuals with celiac sprue develop diarrhea and bloating as young children when they begin to eat cereals, the diagnosis is often missed when inadvertent but therapeutic dietary manipulations, such as elimination diets, are instituted. However, symptoms may improve spontaneously, and patients may appear to "outgrow" the disease until they are in their twenties or thirties. Occasionally latent celiac sprue is activated by a metabolic stress, such as infection, pregnancy, or surgery. Interestingly, about one-quarter of adult-onset sprue patients have a history of diarrhea during childhood.

Celiac sprue is a rare condition. Unless physicians think about it, the patient who presents with the symptoms I have just described is often misdiagnosed as having functional illness, such as irritable bowel syndrome, food allergy, or milk intolerance, or a psychiatric illness.

Once a physician is tenacious enough or perhaps enough of a detective to push further into the realm of the unusual, documenting the presence of celiac sprue is a straightforward task.

A doctor who suspects sprue may ask the patient to collect stool samples to determine whether there is malabsorption of nutrients. Several tests can suggest the diagnosis of celiac sprue. Routine blood testing usually shows anemia and low levels of carotene, cholesterol, iron, calcium, and magnesium. Measurement of blood clotting may be abnormally prolonged as a result of malabsorption of the fat-soluble vitamin K. Occasionally physicians order a xylose tolerance test. For this, patients drink a solution of xylose, a type of sugar, and its absorption is quantified by measuring its concentration in the blood or urine.

More recently, blood tests have been developed that measure antibodies directed against gliadin, the toxic fraction of gluten, as well as against other body constituents, such as smooth muscle cells. Unfortunately, these antibodies may be present in healthy individuals and absent in people with celiac sprue.

Most physicians believe a small intestinal biopsy, a minor surgical procedure, should be performed to document intestinal injury compatible with celiac sprue because of the need for diagnostic certainty before recommending a lifelong change in diet.

Small intestinal biopsies are obtained most often with the use of a fiberoptic endoscope, which is passed into the duodenum after the patient is sedated. A small forceps is passed through the endoscope and multiple biopsies are obtained from the proximal small intestine. Alternately, an intestinal biopsy specimen is obtained with a special-purpose tube passed into the small intestine under X-ray guidance. The biopsy specimens are then carefully oriented and prepared for microscopic examination.

Under the microscope, patients with sprue demonstrate loss of the normal intestinal architecture. In a healthy patient, the intestine consists of innumerable fingerlike projections, called villi, which extend into the intestinal lumen and provide an enormous surface area for absorption. Gluten-induced inflammation leads to the destruction of the lining cells and gradual flattening of the villi until the surface area available for absorption is reduced manyfold.

The most compelling evidence for a correct diagnosis of celiac sprue is the complete disappearance of symptoms on a gluten-free diet. Over a period of weeks to months, the symptoms, signs, and laboratory abnormalities of malabsorption disappear. Patients may feel better within several days of gluten withdrawal, even before the intestinal lesions heal, which suggests that gluten toxicity affects the central nervous system.

The treatment of celiac sprue is straightforward, at least to the physician. Many a patient has heard the words "Just follow a gluten-free diet and you'll be feeling great in a couple of weeks." Unfortunately, many otherwise excellent diagnosticians do not understand the implications, complexities, difficulties, and frustrations encountered in following this simple order.

Other important ancillary measures to reverse the deficiencies caused by malabsorption include multivitamin therapy, including calcium supplements to restore bone density and to facilitate the healing of fractures.

Once they receive the correct diagnosis and adhere to a gluten-free diet, most celiac sprue patients will live a long and happy life. After dealing with the difficulties of living on a gluten-free diet, most patients will cheat occasionally without developing symptoms. Some may do so with great frequency and show no outward signs of recurrence. However, the exposure to gluten leads to subclinical disease. Chronic stimulation of the immune system makes the sprue patient more likely to develop cancer or refractory sprue, a type of sprue that is not affected by a gluten-free diet. The latter condition occurs when scar tissue is laid down in the intestinal wall that prevents proper absorptive function. Once this condition develops, it is largely untreatable, and patients may have to subsist on chronic intravenous feedings. Needless to say, I seriously caution the celiac patient not to compromise this serious condition further by challenging the diet. This introduction should serve as a background to the most important issue facing a celiac sprue patient, "How do I live on a gluten-free diet?" I recommend learning the adaptive behavior presented in this highly entertaining and informative book and challenging oneself to enjoy life to the fullest despite the condition.

Dr. Levine is Head of the Division of Gastroenterology and Nutrition at Albert Einstein Medical Center and Professor of Medicine at Temple University School of Medicine.

Wheat and Food Allergy, Fact and Fiction

Fergus Shanahan, M.D.

A discussion of wheat allergy requires clarification of controversial issues surrounding the more general subject of food allergy. Although the ability of certain foods to trigger allergic reactions in susceptible individuals was convincingly demonstrated more than sixty years ago—long before the modern immunologic era—since then the subject has been shrouded in confusion and controversy. Many physicians approach the subject of food allergy with skepticism. Indeed, some physicians have relegated food allergy to the realm of faddism, cultism, and quackery.

This unfortunate situation has arisen, in part, because of the widespread use of inappropriate terminology and the failure to distinguish food allergy from other forms of adverse reaction to foods or food additives. Confusion and controversy has been further generated by the failure of some enthusiasts to use an objective and scientifically sound approach to the diagnosis of food allergy. This has led to widespread misconceptions regarding the prevalence, scope, and nature of food allergy. Wild and exaggerated accounts of food allergy have appeared in the popular press, generating more public concern for the issue than is warranted and bolstering a public perception that food allergy is a major public health problem. Claims that food allergy can account for disorders as varied as depression, anxiety, fatigue, and obesity have not been scientifically proven and are inappropriate. At the same

7

time, such inaccurate claims have undermined public confidence in the ability of the medical profession to diagnose and treat food allergy.

Fortunately, in the last decade a great deal of scientifically sound work has improved the diagnosis and understanding of *true* food allergy and has returned it to proper perspective.

Recent reviews and recommendations by the American Academy of Allergy and National Institutes of Health have clarified and standardized terminology regarding adverse reactions to food. Similar guidelines have also been produced by the Royal College of Physicians and the British Nutrition Foundation. Adverse reactions to foods may be separated into two broad categories, depending on whether or not the immune system contributes to the abnormal reaction: the term *food allergy* should be reserved for reactions that are mediated by the immune system, whereas the term *food intolerance* refers to all other nonimmunologic reactions to food or food additives. Most adverse reactions to food appear to fall into the nonimmunologic or food intolerance category and are not true allergic disorders. These are highly variable and may be due to toxic or infectious contaminants, or may even be manifestations of underlying gastrointestinal or psychological disorders.

True food allergic reactions may arise as an early reaction (within minutes or hours) or may be delayed (days) after ingestion of a dietary allergen. An example of a delayed response is celiac sprue (also known as gluten-sensitive enteropathy). This is dealt with elsewhere in this book; we will focus on the early allergic reactions here.

Most food allergic reactions are actually caused by a relatively small number of foods. The most commonly implicated food allergens are wheat, milk, eggs, shellfish, soybeans, and nuts. However, it is important to appreciate that various cofactors may contribute to triggering a food allergy or predisposing someone to one. These include exercise after a meal and the ingestion of aspirin or aspirinlike drugs.

The clinical signs and symptoms of food allergy are the same irrespective of which allergen triggers the reaction. However, the severity varies widely in different individuals depending on their allergic susceptibility. Symptoms range in severity from mild, transient discomfort to a life-threatening reaction (referred to as systemic anaphylaxis). The organs most commonly affected are the skin (eczema, itching, urticaria, or hives), the respiratory tract (bronchospasm, "hay-fever"), and the gastrointestinal tract. Gastrointestinal symptoms are non-specific and, depending on the level of the gut primarily affected, range from swelling of the lips to vomiting, cramping, and diarrhea. Studies have shown that food allergy does not appear to be involved in the majority of cases of either irritable bowel syndrome or inflammatory bowel disease. As mentioned earlier, food allergy has been invoked to account for a variety of other disorders without convincing scientific proof.

How common is food allergy? Several studies have shown that there is a discrepancy between perception of food allergy and the results of objective diagnostic tests. Although approximately 20 to 30 percent of adults believe that they have an adverse reaction to some food, the majority of such complaints cannot be verified or reproduced when tested by objective means such as a double-blind food challenge. The estimated prevalence of adverse reactions to foods is less than 2 percent of the adult population, and the likely prevalence of food allergies is probably only a fraction of that overall figure. Food allergy is more common in children and declines with age. It is also more common in individuals with an allergic background, that is, with allergies to other environmental factors such as house dust and pollens. The critical point is that although food allergy is uncommon in adults, it does occur and is a well-documented clinical entity.

When an allergy to wheat or other food is suspected, what is the appropriate method of confirming the diagnosis? Ideally, a certified allergist should be consulted. Objective confirmation of a diagnosis of adverse reaction to food is by an elimination diet, followed by a controlled food challenge, the most definitive evidence being a double-blind food challenge. Evidence that the reaction is immunologically mediated, that is, a true food allergy, can be obtained either by skin testing with the implicated food or by blood tests, which detect antibodies to the food allergen. It is important to recognize that a positive skin test or positive blood test merely demonstrates the presence of antibodies to the implicated food. Many normal or nonallergic individuals have such antibodies. Therefore, without a food challenge, positive results on these antibody tests do not prove that the symptoms are due to an adverse reaction to the food.

In practice, the diagnostic approach to suspected food allergy is individualized and the rigor with which one attempts to prove the diagnosis by a food challenge will be influenced by factors such as the severity of the symptoms and the nutritional importance of the food implicated. In the case of patients with a history of severe reactions or anaphylaxis, further investigations may be unnecessary and potentially dangerous. The implicated food should be avoided and a food challenge or skin test should not be attempted. In contrast, for patients who are thought to be allergic to several major food groups, accurate confirmation of the diagnosis is required because of the inconvenience and danger of malnutrition with prolonged, complicated restriction diets.

It is important to appreciate that food challenges and skin testing with food antigens can trigger potentially serious and even fatal anaphylaxis in a small percentage of patients. Such diagnostic tests should be carried out only by experienced physicians and should be attempted only in a facility equipped to deal with serious allergic reactions. Unfortunately, various unconventional tests for the diagnosis of food allergy have been employed by some enthusiasts. These include the so-called cytotoxicity test. This and other controversial techniques have not withstood rigorous scientific scrutiny and, therefore, are not considered reliable.

The only acceptable form of treatment of food allergy is avoidance of the offending food. Improvements in food labeling requirements with more attention to detail have helped prevent adverse reactions to food and food additives. However, occasional inadvertent ingestion of food allergens should be anticipated. The clear message from documented cases of fatal allergic reactions to food is that patients with a history of severe food allergic reactions should consult an experienced physician, preferably an allergist, and be instructed in self-administration of epinephrine at the first sign of a systemic reaction. For less severe reactions, antihistamine and steroid drugs are sufficient.

Finally, there is the question of prevention of food allergy during childhood. Unfortunately, definitive studies are lacking, but there is some evidence to suggest that breastfeeding until the age of six months may have a protective effect against development of food allergies.

Fergus Shanahan, M.D., is Chairman and Professor of Medicine at the National University of Ireland, Cork University Hospital.

CHAPTER ONE

The Good News. The Bad News.
The Basics.

"Take some more tea," the March Hare said to Alice very earnestly.
"I've had nothing yet," Alice replied in an offended tone; "so I can't take more."
"You mean you can't take less," said The Hatter, "it's very easy
to take more than nothing."

—LEWIS CARROLL
from *Alice's Adventures in Wonderland*

You're not dead. And this is very good news.

Not only are you not dead, you don't have anything that could be vaguely construed as fatal or even remotely life threatening, unless you cheat constantly, and you're not going to do that, are you? You have a disease or an intolerance or, in some cases, an allergy that is managed quite nicely without drugs, doctors, or hospital stays and that does not require that you suffer any more bad news and disquieting symptoms than you already have. Basically, your odd little immune system and the pool from which your particular genes were plucked have tricked your body into thinking bread and other foods considered about as basic to human life as breathing are poison. As I'm sure everyone has told you by now, it could have been worse.

In other words, all the years of mild discomfort, outright pain, unceasing and varied complaints to all manner of exotic medical specialists—most of whom took you seriously and tried to help, while others who shall remain forever in your black book chalked you up to hypochondriacal whining—elimination diets, shots, gastrointestinal emergencies, bloating, diarrhea, weight loss, muscle wasting and worse, are over. Gone. History. *Finito.*

More good news—if you stay on your diet, all those nasty symptoms will disappear and you'll feel great again. And who knows, you may even wind up being like everybody else, except for one tiny detail—you have to follow a diet for life that could turn even the most determined Pollyanna into a vicious serial killer (which, in your case, is spelled *cereal*).

My own case of celiac disease or nontropical sprue—as grain intolerance is referred to in the medical books—took years to discover and a tremendous toll on my health. I suffered mild and seemingly unrelated symptoms all my life without ever getting sick enough to diagnose. At the age of thirty-five, I went into a full-blown celiac syndrome, losing as much as five pounds a week and developing bizarre symptoms, from mysterious and intolerable giant hives to bone pain and a constant low-grade feeling of nausea that seemed to point to very serious disease.

My intestinal villi were so scarred from the offending grain, I had literally stopped absorbing any food and had fallen prey to all kinds of deficiency problems. My hair had completely lost its shine and was falling out in clumps. My muscles had begun to atrophy for lack of protein. I suffered from anemia. Two bones had fractured from lack of calcium absorption, my blood pressure teetered dangerously somewhere around forty over fifty, and I weighed approximately ninety pounds, which at five foot eight, gave me the distinct look of a person wearing someone else's skin. My heart had developed a murmur, I was weak from my frequent trips to the bathroom, and I had to nap in order to recover from the exertion of taking a nap.

When I was finally hauled off to the hospital, all the smart money was on a diagnosis of lymphoma, a cancer of the lymphatic system that reveals itself in many of the same ways as celiac. I was given a bed in a section of the hospital I called the boneyard. Happily, the smart money lost.

Once I was diagnosed, all my past health problems suddenly made sense. My long history of painful and overly long periods was due to my inability to absorb vitamin K, which is necessary in the coagulation of blood. This too was the reason for my puzzling and worrisome resistance to healing. Poor calcium absorption, not a forgotten fall, as one X-ray technician had insinuated, was the reason for the constant pain in my joints. A bone in my right knee and another in my left wrist had developed small atraumatic fractures due to years of constant calcium deprivation. And all the years spent doubled over with what I repeatedly described as the feeling of "glass in my stomach" were not due to a teenager's panic over the SATs or, later, the stress of an advertising career, or a nervous temperament, or PMS, or the push and shove of life in general, or because it was Thursday, or because I was "neurotic," as one baffled diagnostician actually said, playing an especially pernicious form of "blame the victim" when her search for my problem stalled.

In the end, I read the entire physician's diagnostic reference, a door stop of a book called *The Merck Manual,* cross-referencing my symptoms, slogging through the sequelaes, epitheliums, crypts, and lymphocytes with a medical dictionary and a legal pad by my side. When I had my problem narrowed down to the field of gastroenterology, I made an appointment with a superb doctor whose job I made vastly easier by virtue of my self-education—something, incidentally, I advocate for everyone because no one has a better reason to keep trying to find out what's ailing you than you—and together we began the search for the disease that had eluded diagnosis for thirty-five years.

After a series of outpatient tests designed to rule out other serious problems, such as a malfunctioning gall bladder, ulcer, bowel cancer—the usual grizzly suspects—my condition weakened dramatically and it was then I was admitted to Thomas Jefferson Hospital in Philadelphia. There the testing focused on my diminished ability to absorb foods, particularly those with a high fat content, and quickly led to the definitive diagnostic tool, a surgical biopsy. One look at my battered and scarred intestinal villi through his fiber optic viewer and a careful examination of the little snip he took for the lab told my doctor everything he needed to know. I had celiac disease and could thank my father's Irish roots for this peculiar reaction to the gluten found in most grains.

No one really knows why the problem is so much more prevalent in some northern European countries. Legend has it that hundreds and hundreds of years ago, invaders poisoned the wheat harvest. Goths, Huns, the Uncle Ben's people? No one really knows, but as the story goes, over the next several generations the locals adapted by reprogramming their bodies to react to gluten as the poison it was for their ancestors. While it has no basis in scientific fact, I particularly like this theory because it allows me to think I have descended from a fierce and courageous tribe of Gandhi-like people who would not be conquered, adapting instead and becoming the first humans to discover the ultimate power in passive-aggressive behavior.

More good news. The doctor said as long as I lived on a gluten-free diet for the rest of my life, I would be healthy and symptom-free. No medication. No surgery. No medical supervision, except another snip every couple of years to make sure the intestinal wall was healing and there was no new damage. B_{12} shots and megadoses of vitamins were ordered to help speed up my body's badly needed repair.

"Go home, take your supplements, live a normal life," my doctor said, bursting with pride at having detected what lesser physicians usually miss. "Just don't eat any bread, pasta, cookies, sandwiches, tarts, croissants, bagels, granola, bran cereal, cakes, pies, muffins, pastries, sauces, soufflés, stuffing, prepared gravies, crab cakes, pancakes, carrot cakes, chocolate cakes, frozen dinners, canned soups—in fact, most prepared foods—and oh, by the way, Happy Thanksgiving."

It dawned on me very quickly: Life after diagnosis was not going to be a piece of cake. People stared. Waiters glared. Hostesses smiled wanly at my presence at their tables. I became the object of rude questions, questionable dinner conversations, and bad jokes, like "Is a celiac anything like a maniac?" After a while I just stayed home and avoided the whole thing. I didn't know what to do, so I did nothing.

I soon fell victim to what I call the-children-are-starving-in-China syndrome. Everyone around me was profoundly relieved at my diagnosis. I was not going to waste away before their eyes and die of some horrible gastrointestinal cancer. All I had to do was follow a simple diet and I'd be fine. While everyone congratulated themselves on my difficult diagnosis—adult-onset celiac is so much harder to spot than its earlier appearance, usually just after an infant is weaned and put on cereal (I am told babies with gluten intolerance often cling to the bottle as if their little intestines *know*)—my family shed tears of joy and relief, and I suffered an odd form of survivor's guilt, feeling selfish and petty for whining about what seemed like a minor inconvenience in the face of so much real illness in most lives. I wondered what was wrong with me; why I didn't feel as lucky as everyone said I was.

Once my malabsorption problems began to recede and I rose above the wreckage of my physical self, it became clear that I had to make a choice. I could continue to feel sorry for myself and see myself as sick and the focus of a certain amount of negative attention, which for me was an odd mixture of pity and annoyance, or I could turn that attention into a positive and teach myself how to enjoy life again, but not before fully understanding another important piece of news: It's not good news until *you* say it is.

Whether it's wheat allergy or celiac sprue, we all get to diagnosis via a different route. The path is littered with pain and confusion and frustration and angst, but it is also marked by challenge and determination and courage. We have listened to our bodies and persisted despite the fact that our complaints did not fit neatly into one diagnostic drawer or another or stumped people whose specialties were too narrow to include all of our symptoms or whose detective skills were not as sharply honed as we wished them to be.

The truth is, even though it may have taken years or just a few miserable months to figure out the problem, you hung in there and listened to what your body was telling you. You kept pushing, despite the fact that you may have been told more than once that your only problem was your overactive imagination. Your hard-won victory and affirmation of your triumph over illness and suffering needs to be acknowledged. This may come as a surprise to some of you, especially those who were taught to keep a stiff upper lip, but you really don't have to move on just because other people say you do. Whether you have a disease or just an allergy—and we'll talk more later about how damaging the word "just" can be—something very important is missing from your life. It deserves its own mourning period if you are ever to move on.

This really is the first step in healing—being aware of and acknowledging how much it hurt. As I said, with so much real suffering in the world, it is tempting to trivialize a food intolerance, but if you do, you are trivializing yourself and your own sadness and overlooking the basic first step in taking care of yourself—acknowledging the importance of what has just happened to you.

You must tell your story, as I have told you mine, over and over again until you no longer need to tell it. Unfortunately, that may take a little longer than the time allotted to you by others. Never mind. You need to tell it until you can take full credit for getting to this point in your life, for surviving it all, and until you truly believe there is more good news in it than bad.

And there *is* bad news.

You've got something that is not going away, and the wheat- or gluten-free diet you've just been handed is for the rest of your life. You've ordered your last pizza with everything on it and eaten your last double cheeseburger on a sesame seed bun.

So let's get down to basics.

Before you can elaborate on the theme, you have to know the score. You can't be creative about the problem until you know its extent.

Here's the basic gluten-free diet, as it is described in the thirteenth edition of *The Merck Manual* (1977). Incidentally, there is no gluten-free diet in the sixteenth edition (1992). All this later edition says about this difficult diet is that the patient needs "detailed lists of foodstuffs," but it does not say where to obtain them. First piece of basic advice: Run, do not walk, to the nearest registered dietician or nutritionist. Explain it to the HMO later.

GLUTEN-FREE DIET

Indications: Primary malabsorption syndrome (nontropical sprue, celiac disease).

Principle: Elimination of cereal protein, gluten, from the diet by omitting all foods containing wheat, rye, oats, buckwheat, and barley and their derivatives.

Type of Food	Yes Foods	No Foods
Beverage	Carbonated beverages, cocoa powder, tea, coffee, milk	Cereal beverages; cocoa mixes; malted milks, drinks made with malt or other excluded cereals; ale, beer
Bread	Bread and muffins made with arrowroot, corn, potato, rice, or soybean flour	Any made with wheat, barley, rye, or oat flour; crackers, rusk; pretzels, pancakes, prepared mixes
Cereal	Ready-to-eat corn and rice cereals, cornmeal, rice, and hominy	Any made with wheat, oats, rye, bran, malt flavoring, barley, buckwheat, macaroni, noodles, spaghetti
Dessert	Blancmange, custards and puddings made with allowable flours or starches; gelatin desserts; sherbet; tapioca; homemade ice cream; special cookies made without wheat, rye, or oat flour	Any containing wheat, rye, barley, or oat products, such as commercial cakes, cookies, ice cream, pastries, pies, puddings, or those made from commercial mixes.
Fat	Butter, margarine, pure mayonnaise, cooking oils, shortening	Commercial salad dressings, wheat germ oil
Fruit	Any	None
Meat, Egg, or Cheese	Any meat, fish, or fowl except those excluded; natural cheese, eggs	Meat, fish, or chicken or croquettes made with bread or bread crumbs; cheese spreads; canned meat dishes, cold cuts unless pure meat; bread stuffings; gravy thickened with flour

Type of Food	Yes Foods	No Foods
Soup	Broth or bouillon; vegetable soup and cream soups made from allowable foods, thickened with cornstarch or potato flour only	Any containing excluded flours or starches (See p. 36 for further discussion of the prevalence of gluten in commercial soups.)
Sweets	Any except those prepared with excluded grain products	Candy containing wheat, rye, oats, barley
Vegetable	Any except those prepared with excluded grain products	
Miscellaneous	Salt, spices, vinegar,* herbs, pickles, baking chocolate, olives, nuts, peanut butter	All gravies or sauces thickened with wheat flour; flavoring syrups, bottled meat sauces, malt extract

*Even though white vinegar contains wheat, it is believed the distilling process destroys gluten's ability to do harm to all but the most wheat-sensitive people. I say, why push it? Use gluten-free apple cider vinegar, wine vinegar, balsamic vinegar, or rice vinegar in recipes and salads to be on the safe side. They taste much better too.

The American Dietetic Association elaborates on this bare-bones diet, adding Sealtest, Breyer's, and Schrafft's ice creams, fruit whips, and meringues; popcorn; potato chips; Fritos; chocolate; and yogurt to the list of allowable, gluten-free desserts and snacks. Rice, potato, and lima bean flours and wheat-free starch are added to the ingredients in gluten-free breads, rolls, and muffins. The association warns us to read the labels on instant coffee and cocoa products to make sure no wheat flour has been added in the manufacturing process.

Specific no-nos include Postum and other coffee substitutes, Ovaltine, graham flours, Ry-Krisp, waffles, Zwieback, matzo meal, commercial yeast, quick bread mixes, any cereal containing malt flavoring or extract, such as Rice Krispies and most commercial puddings. The association welcomes questions and will send a sample gluten-free diet.

More no-nos:

Forget the so-called "new grains," millet, spelt, and kamut, on the gluten-free diet. The jury is still out on quinoa. Some say yes; some say no. Let your individual sensitivity and your doctor be your guide. Because so little research has been conducted on these unfamiliar grains, the U.S.A. Celiac Sprue Association recommends that people with celiac sprue avoid them. Bleu cheese, Stilton, Gorgonzola, and other veined cheeses are also off-limits for some sensitive types because rumor has it that bread is involved in making the original molds from which the cheese is cultured. Since these secret recipes are more closely guarded than the Pentagon, it's best to avoid the whole thing.

Forget processed cheeses and spreads (which may contain gluten that is not disclosed on the label), vanilla extract, some curry powders, bottled meat sauces, some soy sauces, prepared ketchup, prepared mustard, prepared horseradish (these last three contain white vinegar), MSG, some jelly candies (those containing barley water or that use sugar with barley water for coating), and licorice. Yes, believe it or not, licorice.

Hydrolyzed vegetable protein, vegetable protein, hydrolyzed plant protein, and modified food starch are all in the questionable category, and, as strange as this may sound, not all turkeys are gluten-free. It's not because the turkey may have eaten wheat in his or her lifetime, but because prebasted turkeys and other poultry products, such as Butterball brand, may contain gluten in the "butter" mixture injected into the bird.

Watch those cooking sprays. They contain grain alcohol.

Many candy bars are not gluten-free. Why? It's not because they contain undisclosed wheat-based ingredients, but because wheat flour often is used on the gooey bars to keep them from sticking to each other on the conveyor belts and gumming up the works. This is why some Mars bars, among other brands, are gluten-free and some are not; one factory uses flour in the process and another does not. How do you know? You don't. No law says a food manufacturer must disclose what is *on* the product, only what's *in* it.

What's a consumer to do? Memorize these basic rules:

Basic Rule No. 1

Never forget that you are the customer, and, as such, you are entitled to a complete explanation of a food manufacturer's process.

Remember, without you, companies are out of business. They are not doing you a favor by answering your questions and/or complaints. They want you to tell them what you think. That's why they put their names and addresses so prominently on their packages. I once wrote to a certain prune company and told them what I thought of their pitting machine, enclosing the pit I found in the box that said *pitted*. I don't think I'll be able to eat all the free fruit in this lifetime.

If you really love a product and are not sure how it's made, call, write, or fax the manufacturer's customer service department and find out. If they give you a hard time, tell them you and your friends and your family and everyone you know in this life and the next will boycott their products for all time. If you're up to it, mention that you got very sick eating something the company made. Nobody wants to lose a customer or face a lawsuit for misleading information.

All of which leads to . . .

Basic Rule No. 2

Read labels carefully. Never eat a meal or a packaged food if you don't know what's in it. If there's no label, ask for it. If it's not available, don't risk it.

This rule can be a problem on airlines, at salad bars and catered affairs, and in chain restaurants, fast food establishments, school cafeterias, and weight-loss programs such as Jenny Craig, Nutri/System, and others that sell their frozen meals and diet products directly to clients. Such programs are not required by law to disclose any nutritional information, including calorie and fat content and ingredients, which is why I believe so many people fail on the plans and regain the weight. They have no idea what they've been eating and the minute they resume eating normal food, they overeat.

The point is, whenever you are a captive audience—where you have not specifically requested a gluten-free meal, the chef is unavailable for consultation, or the ingredient label is missing—you are in real danger of consuming hidden gluten. Don't risk it.

Basic Rule No. 3
Don't expect a "miracle" cure.

My doctor told me of another patient of his who continued to suffer symptoms even though she followed the gluten-free diet scrupulously. Just as more tests were being ordered, the devout Catholic woman volunteered that she attended Mass and took Communion every day. Bingo! The wafer used in many Christian services is not gluten-free.

I've got to believe passing up this ritual won't ruin your chances at heaven, but consuming it could make your life "diet hell." By all means, explain your special problem to the pastor. If real wine and a chunk of bread is offered during the service, take the wine and signal "no thanks" by tilting your head down when the priest offers the bread, or just take it, put it in your pocket, and feed the birds. While the church may be able to order gluten-free bread or even a gluten-free wafer, it isn't really practical unless many people in the congregation have the same problem. I figure it this way: If the Big Guy/Gal doesn't know you've got a problem, who does?

If you must have your own wafer, look up the American Celiac Society Dietary Support Coalition in chapter 12 and write for the recipe one of their members developed.

Some other little-known facts:

Licking the gluten problem will not always be easy because the glue used on many envelopes, stamps, and mailing labels contains wheat. Since glue is not a food to most of us over the age of four, this source is easily overlooked. It pays to use a sponge, buy only self-adhering products, ask for the new self-sticking U.S. postage stamps, or forget the whole thing and hire a secretary.

Sniffing glue can be a problem too, and I don't mean the dangerous kind that is against the law and stupid. It is possible to inhale
gluten inadvertently through furniture refinishers or craft kits, paste
wax, and the like. Try to avoid using these substances. If you must, use
them infrequently and in a well-ventilated area. I am allergic to dust
mites as well as to gluten, so I play it safe when digging around in
dusty closets or working with paste wax and glue. I wear a surgical
mask, which is available in most drugstores. Remember, though, to
slip it off before answering the doorbell. The last time I forgot, the
post person apologized for interrupting me in the middle of surgery
and asked how the patient was doing.

The term *grain alcohol* should tell you all you need to know about
drinking beer, ale, rye, malt, and Scotch whiskey blends, including
corn whiskey, which uses grain mash. Bourbons, Canadian blends, and
most liqueurs are off-limits too. Rum and tequilla are safe, and vodka
is gluten-free, as long as it is made from potatoes—not grain, which
sadly is the case with many vodkas on the market today.

On the plus side, a trip to wine country will be a special joy for
the gluten-impaired, because pure wine, from the mellow Merlots to
the crisp Chardonnays and all the varieties in between, is mercifully
gluten-free. This includes sherries, ports, cognacs, brandies, and saki,
the Japanese rice wine. As with everything, though, read the label.
Distilleries sometimes substitute wheat in the process and use preservatives and additives, just as food manufacturers do.

Basic Rule No. 4
*If you don't understand it, don't eat it until you do. If you can't remember,
carry a cheat sheet to the supermarket.*

This is one time ignorance is not bliss. Anyway, it's embarrassing
to have spent your hard-earned money on foods that are keeping you
sick. Let's review some basic food additives.

Hydrolyzed vegetable protein, vegetable protein, or **hydrolyzed plant protein.** Often abbreviated HVP or HPP on food
labels, these additives commonly are made from wheat or wheat

mixed with corn or soy. If you know for sure a particular protein is made from corn or soy only, it's safe to eat.

Malt or malt flavoring. All usually are made from barley malt or syrup and are often found in cereals, cookies, and candies. They are not gluten-free.

Modified food starch or **modified starch.** These starches commonly are made from corn and sometimes from arrowroot, potato, or tapioca, but also from wheat. If you can be certain which ingredient went into the product you are considering, *bon appétit.*

Starch. When you see simply "starch" listed on a manufacturer's label, it means it is made from cornstarch only, in keeping with an FDA requirement.

Vegetable gums. Be careful to avoid any product that contains oat gum. If a vegetable gum is made from carob bean, guar gum, gum arabic, gum acacia, locust bean, cellulose gum, gum tragacanth or just plain gum, while it may sound unpalatable, it isn't.

Basic Rule No. 5
It's better to look silly than to get sick. Remember, there are worse things to be called than "fussy."

Only a crumb would ask you to share a toaster. This may sound like Felix's fuddy-duddy behavior in the *The Odd Couple,* but Newton's law of physics makes a toaster oven a better choice than a conventional toaster because it allows your bread to toast flat, clear of the crumbs that normally drop off breads, muffins, and bagels and collect on the bottom, mixing with your gluten-free bread. After I explained my theory of "crumb contamination" to the person who sold me my toaster oven, the speed with which I was served and shown the door set a record for that small-appliance store chain.

Basic Rule No. 6
Make sure you know who or what is touching your food at all times.

People can spread gluten just like viruses, and, in fact, you can make yourself sick by not washing your hands after handling wheat flour. Watch inanimate sources of contagion too, such as deep-fat fryers and grills, either in restaurants or in your own backyard. If they're not scraped carefully, they could contaminate your food.

Find out if a restaurant uses its fryer for breaded dishes as well as for French fried potatoes and if its griddle is reasonably clean and scraped after each use. If the grill is in plain sight, watch the cook prepare a few orders and see for yourself or get up and walk right into the kitchen or ask the owner for a tour. No need to be shy. (More about this necessary skill in chapter 5.) Obviously, you're not going to do this in a truck stop or a coffeeshop you'll never see again, but it is very important to establish your needs in a restaurant you frequent often, particularly one near your office or workplace. Home or a barbecue with friends is easy. Just make sure your food is first up on the backyard grill.

Right about now, you're asking "Will I ever eat again?" The answer is yes, and you will eat more than you ever dreamed because I will tell how to get what you want and where to look for it. But first you need to learn how to stock the basic pantry, which you will eventually tailor to your own tastes and living habits, adding and subtracting the ingredients and staples you need to keep on hand for the ideas you'll find in subsequent chapters. (Hint: You're not going to need a pasta machine if you're too busy working to make your bed.)

The well-rounded wheat- and gluten-free pantry includes the following basics.

Arrowroot. This thickening agent blends well with most wheat- and gluten-free flours and makes a great turkey gravy.

Brown and white rice flours. Keep these on hand and use them for dusting, dredging, flouring hands, and mixing with other gluten-free flours for cooking and baking.

Cereals. Breakfast is no longer "grab a piece of toast, a roll, or a Danish and dash," so always keep a box of gluten-free cold cereal, hominy grits, and hot rice cereal on the shelf. It's a good idea to keep individual boxes of cold cereal at the office or in your work bag as well. You never know when the alarm clock will fail you and leave no time for breakfast. I add my own nuts and raisins, which are fresher and tastier than those rock-hard "droppings" that pass for fruit in cereals these days.

Corn flour. This silky version of cornmeal is the right texture for corn muffins and other baked goods or recipes requiring a lighter result than cornmeal alone can achieve.

Cornmeal. You'll need to keep this staple on hand for cereals, crusts, accompaniments to roasts, soft or grilled polenta, and gluten-free batters. Corn bread makes an excellent addition to stuffings, meat loaf, and other ground meat dishes and can often replace bread crumbs in standard recipes.

Cornstarch. Like arrowroot, this is a great thickening agent for sauces and gravies and is less prone to lumps than wheat flour.

Exotic flours. You may want to keep on hand small amounts of unusual flours made from lentils, peas, artichokes, acorns, beans, mung beans, chick peas, almonds, hazelnuts, and pistachios, but unless you are going to use them consistently, they are best bought fresh. It is best to buy nuts for nut flours—used in many "flourless" cake and torte recipes—as you need them, and then to grind them yourself, as the high oil content tends to turn rancid when stored for long periods.

Gluten-free breads. These are available in health food stores and by mail (see chapter 12). By the time you finish this book, you will have a million uses for them. Many of these breads are sold in shelf-stable packages and, for this reason, can be ordered in quantity. Most breads freeze well, so keep yourself stocked.

Gluten-free pastas. Yes, Virginia, there is a Santa Claus, and he is Italian. More about that in chapter 2.

Oriental rice sticks and noodles. These are available in Asian markets and health food stores and require very little preparation, usually no more than soaking, for use in gluten-free cooking.

Potato flour. Don't confuse this with potato starch flour. Potato flour is made from the whole potato. A small amount goes a long way to refine the texture of the grainier rice flours. For example, 1 teaspoon potato flour is enough to redefine the texture of ½ cup rice flour, or as little as 1 tablespoon can retexturize 1 or 2 cups rice flour.

Potato starch flour. This thickener is interchangeable with cornstarch and can be found in most supermarkets or health food stores.

Rices. Stock up on white rice, brown rice, wild rice, sweet Basmati rice, Arborio, and all the gorgeous varieties of this delicious grain you can afford. If you're like me, you'll find yourself developing a new appreciation for this ubiquitous and gluten-free staple.

Soy or soya flour. As this can have a heavy flavor when used alone, it should be used in conjunction with other milder flours. Since it is high in fat and protein, it can add nutrients and needed moisture to an otherwise dry recipe. For example, if a recipe calls for 2 cups wheat flour, use 1 cup rice flour, ¾ cup potato starch flour, and ¼ cup soy flour.

Sweet rice flour. This is usually found in Asian food markets and health food stores. Because it has more starch than regular rice flour, it makes an excellent thickening agent.

Tapioca flour. Use this flour in recipes where a light texture is required, as in pancakes and waffles. It is on a par with and, in some cases, superior to wheat flour.

Xanthan gum. This is used as a binder, thickener, or stabilizer. It is used commercially as a suspension agent in salad dressings and in pie fillings, canned gravies, and sauces to give these products a smoother texture. It is made by using the bacteria *Xanthomonas compestris* to ferment corn sugar. If you are planning to bake your own gluten-free breads and baked goods, you'll need to stock up on it.

NOTE: All flours and meals should be tightly sealed and kept in the refrigerator to avoid rancidity and mealybugs. Most freeze well and can be kept for months this way. Date everything you freeze. If you're like me, you'll forget when you put it in faster than ice can form.

Is the gluten-free diet tax deductible? The Internal Revenue Service Taxpayer Hot Line says "Yes!—*if* you have a note from your doctor describing your disease and clearly stating that gluten-free foods are necessary for the maintenance of your health . . . and *if* you have itemized deductions exceeding $300 in 1994."

Subtract the cost of the "normal" product from the higher price of the gluten-free product and deduct the difference. Of course, anything can be challenged, so in case of an audit, your accountant or the person who prepares your taxes needs to understand and support the necessity of this deduction in order to defend it properly.

Another word of advice. Get thee to a dietitian. Better, a registered dietitian who can assess the nutritional damage, design a program for healthy eating and achieving normal weight, and help you heal and stay that way. For referrals, contact the American Dietetic Association listed in chapter 12.

Remember that there is always safety *and* support in numbers. Join a national organization and get on the gluten-free grapevine with newsletters, recipes, medical information, the latest on ingredient labeling, medical research, associated problems, diagnosis, local support groups, and gluten-free gatherings complete with speakers, product demonstrations, entertainment, new product sampling, and the potential for some new pals.

A valuable resource, especially for the latest medical research and diagnostic information, is the Celiac Disease Foundation. Write Elaine Monarch and ask for their nutritional guidelines as well as for a "starter packet" of information that includes sources for gluten-free foods. Don't forget to get their button, "Celiacs do it gluten-free." I consider mine a walking ad for awareness of grain intolerance and wear it in my baseball cap, happily enlightening all who ask.

Other worthwhile support groups are the Celiac Sprue Association/United States of America (based in Omaha), Gluten Intolerance Group of North America (Seattle), American Celiac Society Dietary Support Coalition (New Jersey), the American Allergy Association (California), and the Canadian Celiac Association. They are all listed in chapter 12, along with names and addresses for local support groups in your area.

A final bit of basic advice. Never join the first club you call. Make sure the organization you choose shares your goals and can help you achieve them. Call them all and decide which one feels right for you.

CHAPTER TWO

Marketing 101

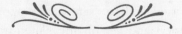

Caveat emptor.
—Proverb

Armed with the basic knowledge of what you can and what you can't eat and assuming you are no longer wearing a hospital gown and paper slippers and trailing an intravenous tube, you are now ready for your next big adventure—grocery shopping. And believe me, if you don't do your homework properly, the expression "Shop till you drop" is a lot closer to the truth than you think.

The Supermarket

Think of your local supermarket as a giant chemistry lab where better living and longer shelf life are achieved through additives, stabilizers, fillers, emulsifiers, preservatives, artificial colors, flavors, fats, and gums made of dubious and arcane ingredients. Despite packaging that would have you believe otherwise, you are surrounded by foods that have been processed into nutritional hell and bear only a passing resemblance to the ones that occur in nature. Further, there is no kindly grocer; no one, for that matter, who is able to answer your questions.

You find yourself at the mercy of sullen part-timers, truants, baggers, and stock clerks who seriously believe Frito trees are why we should save the rain forests. Your mere presence in this hotbed of hidden wheat- and gluten-based ingredients could seriously compromise your health, not to mention your good standing in Greenpeace. What *is* guar gum, anyway?

> GUAR GUM: According to *Webster's New Collegiate Dictionary*, guar gum is "a gum that consists of the ground endosperm of guar seeds and is used especially as a thickening agent and sizing material." Endosperm, as everyone knows, is a nutritive tissue on seed plants formed within the embryo sac. Basically, this is the stuff used on your sheets and shirts to make them feel crisp. Eat as much as you like; guar gum is gluten-free.
>
>

In situations like this, it helps to think of yourself as a kind of grain Geiger counter, quietly ticking around the perimeter of the store, where fresh meats, produce, dairy, deli, and bakery products are found, getting louder as you move toward the aisles on either side, going full tilt as you find yourself in Soups, Hamburger Helpers, and Dips, losing its little mind in Pastas, Cereals, and Snacks.

A good rule to remember is the more processed the product, the more risk it contains for you. And conversely, the fresher the food, the better your chances of being able to eat it. I also have found there is a strong correlation between convenience and gluten. Those fast and costly little dinner trays collecting ice crystals in your freezer offer no relief in the convenience food category. Sadly, most frozen entrées and side dishes are so loaded with gluten as to be inedible, but this will take awhile to sink in. Until it does, you will stare endlessly through a fog of condensation and your own regrets, like some poor exile to the Gulag, as other people open and close the doors, filling their carts with goodies until you are satisfied there is nothing much in there for you, except Breyers ice cream and Green Giant frozen peas. By all means, stand there and read every label until you have seen this for yourself, but do wear a sweater and gloves. The thought of a cold without chicken noodle soup is too sad to contemplate.

As you consider your old friend the supermarket in the new light of your diet, try to remember these simple rules.

1. It is always better to buy the ingredients and assemble a meal yourself than to buy one that has already been boxed, bagged, canned, hermetically sealed, or rendered shelf stable by someone on an assembly line. (The truth is, it's just as easy to bake or broil a chicken breast as it is to warm one that is already cooked, sauced and full of gluten, calories, and chemicals. If it's any consolation, it's also cheaper and less fattening.)

2. Buy one of those coupon organizers. Add a list of wheat- and gluten-free products to each section along with the appropriate cents-off coupons. You're already paying through your stomach, why pay through the nose too?

3. What you can't read *can* hurt. If you have trouble reading the small print on any packaged food, even when held at arm's length, never enter a supermarket without your glasses or, for a more dramatic statement, a small magnifying glass. Wear these things on a ribbon around your neck so you always know where they are and you can take them on and off easily to prevent eye strain.

4. Just as the words *fat-free* scrawled across a package do not mean calorie-free, *wheat-free* and *all natural* do not necessarily mean *gluten-free*. Remember, people who want you to buy their products, not the FDA, design packages. Always read the fine print. And speaking of reading . . .

5. Do your homework at home. Lighting and other conditions conducive to reading are not exactly ideal in a supermarket aisle and, at peak shopping times, may even be considered a form of public torture. The more you know ahead of time, the faster it will go. The less time spent rubbing carts with people who are loading up on cookies, coffee cake, and bagels, the better. Remember, it is not considered attractive to drool over other people's groceries.

You should be able to execute a wheat- and gluten-free run to the market fairly easily and without undue delays, once you know what

you're looking for. Products and conditions will vary according to regional tastes and from store to store, and product formulations may
change with no warning. (Always check with the manufacturer if you
really want to be sure.) Here's a typical aisle-by-aisle assessment of
availability based on my own neighborhood Pathmark, a typical supermarket chain store in the Northeast, product information supplied
by the Celiac Sprue Association/USA and the food makers themselves.
Understand that ingredients change and food companies may change
them without reprinting their labels. The products mentioned here as
wheat- and/or gluten-free have been declared such by their makers,
either by virtue of their package labels or through customer service
inquiries, and are such to the best of my knowledge at this printing.
Always call and check before you stock up on something you like or
try something you're not sure of.

DIET PRODUCTS

If you don't want to lose twenty pounds in twenty minutes, this
aisle is a real danger zone. Avoid concoctions like those made by Slim
Fast and Nestlé. Only a chemist could be sure of the ingredients in the
drinks, and the powders usually contain malt extract and maltodextrin,
among other dubious grain derivatives. If you must lose weight this
way, discuss it with your doctor first and do not begin until you are
positive the product you are using contains no wheat or gluten. For
the names, addresses, and toll-free numbers of these and other food
marketers mentioned in this section, refer to chapter 12.

DRUGS

Read the labels of all cold, allergy, sinus, and flu medications very
carefully. Many medications sold in the United States contain no
wheat or gluten, but if you want more tangible proof, contact the FDA
or the drug company for the definitive analysis or write to Celiac
Sprue Association/USA for a comprehensive drug information guide.
Another route is to invest in your own *Physicians' Desk Reference* ($64.95
for the 1995 edition), which is revised every year and lists nearly all
manufactured pharmaceutical prescription products in the United
States, dosage instructions, precautions, contraindications, and all
ingredients. Or better, borrow your pharmacist's copy or look it up

in the library. A companion edition, *Physician's Desk Reference for Non-Prescription Drugs*, lists all over-the-counter medications, provides toll-free numbers for each manufacturer, and costs $41.95 for the 1995 edition. Add $5.95 shipping and handling per book. See "Required Reading," page 255, for ordering information.

Watch out for patent medicines, such as antacids, laxatives, and cough syrups, and simple, everyday products such as toothpaste. Contact big players—Procter & Gamble, Rhone-Poulenc, Colgate Palmolive, Cheesebrough Pond's, and Arm & Hammer—regarding the wheat- and gluten-free status of your favorite brand. The only other alternative is to get a postgraduate degree in chemistry before your next case of heartburn.

Don't think you are home free in cosmetics either. Many talcums, body powders, shampoos, and hand creams contain gluten and may cause symptoms in extremely sensitive individuals.

Unless you are planning to drink the water from your washer's rinse cycle, spin through detergents, bleaches, fabric softeners, and ditto for cling wraps, storage bags, tin foil, waxed paper, surface cleaners, automotive supplies, and stationery, but watch out for the glue on those stamps and envelopes.

BAKING NEEDS

General Foods lists Calumet baking powder as gluten-free. While most buttered syrups are to be avoided, Quaker Oats claims its Aunt Jemima Original syrup is gluten-free as does Kraft/General Foods of its Log Cabin syrup. And of course pure maple syrup is gluten-free. Read labels on all prepared mixes very carefully, but look for Manischewitz wheat- and gluten-free potato pancake and kugel mixes, Penn Foods potato dumpling and pancake mixes, Quaker corn flour, and rice and potato products from Fearn, Elam's, and Featherweight. These claim to be wheat- and gluten-free.

Nestlé's and Hershey's chocolate morsels are deemed safe by their makers for use in the gluten-free baking mixes and pie shells discussed later. Don't forget to pick up cornmeal in this aisle. You'll use it for coatings, polenta, corn cakes, fried chicken, corn bread, and cornmeal mush. General Foods claims it has rendered its Stovetop Cornbread Stuffing gluten-free in the flexible serving size only.

Avert your eyes in the cake mix section and try not to breathe in the gluten as you pass those dusty sacks of flour. Procter & Gamble's Duncan Hines Chocolate Frosting, Dark Dutch Fudge Frosting, Milk Chocolate Frosting, and Vanilla Frosting all claim to be gluten-free. Remember, ingredients often vary with flavors, so read every label carefully. Avoid flavored extracts. They are not gluten-free.

MEATS

The rule here is simple. If it comes from a fairly recognizable part of a cow, sheep, pig, or chicken and nothing has been added, it's okay to eat. If the meat in question is preserved in any way or is an unspecified blend of animal and other ingredients, such as those found in hot dogs, it is usually not gluten-free. The exceptions are Kosher all-beef cocktail frankfurters, Oscar Mayer beef franks and cheese dogs, and some sausages and other ground meat products whose manufacturers claim contain no cereal fillers or that list the products to be wheat- and gluten-free on the label. If the cereal fillers and stabilizers don't get you, the sodium and nitrates will. It's not worth the trouble. If you must buy this stuff, call the company before you do.

Armour and Rath canned hams, Spam, and Swanson's canned chicken, turkey, and chunks o' chicken are gluten-free. Never buy scrapple, a Pennsylvania Dutch regional breakfast food made of pig scraps and other unspecified animal and vegetable bits. It's full of wheat flour and is gray when cooked. Enough said?

Be wary of prebasted birds. The basting mixture may contain wheat, which bothers many grain-sensitive people. Also, be careful when buying premarinated meat and fish steaks (the marinade may contain soy sauce, mustard, or vinegar), prestuffed pork chops, or premixed meat loaf or any convenience meats. Consider the prices of these goodies versus the unadorned varieties and ask yourself, "How lazy can I get?"

COOKIES AND SNACKS

The skimpy selection of rice cakes isn't worth the pain of stopping in this aisle chock full of memories of Mallowmars and Oreos. My personal fantasy is to wake up one day and find out R. J. R. Nabisco has plowed all its cigarette profits into research to develop the world's first gluten-free Oreo. Keep moving.

Speaking of snacks, I ran into the Best Foods representative one day while I was squinting hard at a Skippy Peanut Butter label in a South Philadelphia Pathmark. When I spotted him, I was delighted to be able to ask him who at Best Foods could best translate their label to me. He glazed over, stepped back as if I might have a contagious disease, and refused to give it to me, telling me that information was confidential, even after I informed him that most companies print their phone numbers right on their packages for customers to call with questions. He ended the conversation by saying, "I hope you under-stand. We have to protect ourselves."

"From whom?" I asked. "Your customers?" I really wanted to run him over with my shopping cart and tell him to stick *that* on the roof of his mouth, but I resisted the impulse. Instead I smiled sweetly and said quite calmly, "I'll bet if I got sick and died from eating Skippy Peanut Butter, my lawyer could find that number."

Face it now, this is going to happen to you too. We are a litigious society, and people will mistrust your motive for asking about their ingredients. Never just skulk away and buy another brand. Always let the offending company know, preferably within earshot of other cus-tomers, why you are doing business with someone else.

Console yourself with popcorn, Cracker Jacks, Fiddle Faddle, and Fritos. They all claim to be gluten-free. Beware of Cheetos, which contain gluten, not listed on the label.

Canned Goods

Most Bush's baked beans contain starch from an undisclosed source. B & M brand baked beans contain mustard (a no-no because it could contain white vinegar). Heinz Vegetarian Baked Beans and Hunt's Big John's Beans and Fixin's contain vinegar of an unspecified nature. Campbell's Pork 'n Beans contain modified food starch and vin-egar. If you love them, as I do occasionally, baked to a satisfying sticki-ness with a hefty pork chop, it pays to contact the company for the final word. Hunt's Pork & Beans, Bush's Deluxe Pork and Beans, Hunt's Original Manwich and Mexican Manwich, and Allen's Baked Beans are all listed as gluten-free.

All plain canned beans are wheat- and gluten-free. People like us tend to "gurgle," so don't forget to pick up some Beano, an antiflatulent, and enjoy your beans quietly.

CONDIMENTS, COCKTAIL SAUCES, AND DRESSINGS

Hellman's Mayonnaise, both Regular and Light, is gluten-free, but most mustards are not because they contain vinegar, which could be white. A call to Nabisco, the makers of Grey Poupon, assured me that my favorite mustard is gluten-free. Contact with French's or Gulden's or whoever makes your favorite is certainly worth the effort for the final word on this ubiquitous and fat-free dressing.

Sadly, the big makers of barbecue sauce and ketchup—Kraft, Heinz, Hunt's, and Con Agra (Healthy Choice)—use vinegar, mustard, and/or mustard flour in their products, but General Foods' Open Pit Barbecue sauces claims to be gluten-free in all varieties, as does Hunt's All Natural Barbecue Sauce and Meatloaf Fixin's Tomato Sauce.

Newman's Own Salad Dressing is not only very good in Regular or Light, but is said to be wheat- and gluten-free. I might add that this is the socially conscious choice as well, in that a percentage of the profits from all of Paul Newman's products goes to wonderful charities. Pour some of his good dressing into any small sterile bottle or clean plastic container with a tight lid to take to restaurants, to the office, and on vacation. And don't worry. Under the circumstances, it's politically correct to carry salad dressing in one's pocket.

If you like to mix your own, General Foods Good Seasons Salad Dressing mixes are said to be gluten-free in all but the Bleu Cheese and Herbs and Cheese Garlic varieties. Ditto for Lawry's mixes in Italian and Italian with cheese.

HEALTH FOODS

This tiny corner in my supermarket manages to hold not one but three kinds of cookies—Nature's Warehouse wheat-free cookies, Pamela's gluten-free shortbread cookies, and Cathy's wheat-free fig bars. More about these goodies later.

Also found in this small but satisfying section are Mother's Rice and Popcorn Cakes, Hain rice and popcorn minicakes, and Guiltless Gourmet fat-free tortilla chips and salsa. Watch out for the fat-free bean dips and fat-free nacho cheese dips. These contain vinegar. Don't forget to scour the Hispanic Foods section for a bigger selection of salsas and corn products.

SOUPS

The bad news is that most canned soups, especially cream soups, are mmmm-bad for people like us. Gluten and wheat can't hide in anything clear, so if you love broths and bouillons, the good news is you'll be eating quite a bit of them from now on, but don't trust them all. Read every label individually.

Among those declared wheat- and gluten-free by their companies are Campbell's Split Pea with Ham, Hearty Lentil, and Country Vegetable. Oyster stew from Chicken of the Sea, and beef liver and chicken from Heinz have also been given the company okay.

Vichyssoise, Crab, and Chicken with Wild Rice gourmet soups from Pepperidge Farm contain yeast extract, that frothy stuff that causes breads to rise and can cause reactions in those sensitive to it, but otherwise they appear to be wheat- and gluten-free. Write these companies for the definitive word and a complete list of products.

TOPPINGS, PUDDINGS, JAMS, AND BEVERAGES

I prefer melting good chocolate and pouring it directly over my ice cream if I am in the mood for a high-fat splurge, but those of you who have fond memories of chocolate syrup should be advised that Smucker's Fudge Syrup contains food starch, which could be wheat based and its Sundae Syrup contains food starch and oat flour.

Hershey's Chocolate Milk Mix and Nestlé Quick contain malto-dextrin, but Sugar-free Quick and Cocoa Mix appear to be wheat-free. If you are going to suffer as a result of having sworn off this stuff, it really is worth the trouble to call or write Smucker's or Hershey's first to find out what kind of food starch is used.

Jell-O Americana Golden Egg Custard Mix, Rice Pudding, and Tapioca puddings, Minute Tapioca, and Jell-O Rich & Luscious Mousse mixes are listed as gluten-free by their maker, General Foods. Also declared gluten-free are D-Zerta, reduced calorie and regular, and sugar-free Jell-O puddings and pie fillings. Instant varieties are not.

Most Snack Pack pudding flavors from Hunt's are gluten-free as are Nabisco Royal puddings, Salada Danish dessert mixes, My-T-Fine lemon and tapioca, and Delmonte and Betty Crocker puddings.

Swiss Miss Cocoa Mixes, Cocoa with Mini Marshmallows, Milk Chocolate, Double Rich Hot Cocoa, Lite, and Sugar-Free varieties are all listed as gluten-free. Nestlé's Carnation Rich Chocolate flavor instant breakfast is wheat-free only.

Read the labels on all beverage mixes and be careful in the coffee section. Ground coffee beans are fine, but some instant brews are made with cereal. All International coffees from General Foods, both sugar-free and sugar sweetened, are said to be gluten-free except Café Vienna and Orange Cappuccino. Nondairy creamers from Borden's, Carnation, Dewey Fresh, and Rich's Coffee Rich are all on the allowed list.

THE FREEZER CASE

Basically all plain frozen vegetables are okay, but watch out for any frozen vegetable or side dishes with sauce. Many contain wheat flour or wheat starch as a thickening agent. Keep walking past frozen dinners, bagels, and frozen pies and cakes. Forget fancy toaster products too. This is the "post–Pop Tart" age. Slow down when you get to ice cream and frozen desserts. Breyers, Sealtest and Schrafft's have been declared by their makers to be gloriously gluten-free.

Ben & Jerry's Homemade proclaims all natural ingredients as well, but because of their exotic mixtures, each flavor must be examined very carefully, and a follow-up call to the boys in Vermont would not hurt at all. My own call to Vermont elicited concern regarding extracts, which are purchased as commodities and do not always come from the same source, and a serious interest in finding alternative, gluten-free sources. (Ben or Jerry: See chapter 4!)

Häagen-Dazs also declares itself "all natural." Call them for the flavor you may be able to enjoy safely. Remember our friend The Mad Hatter: "Better to take less than nothing at all."

General Foods Jell-O Fruit Bars, Gelatin, and Pudding Pops, Cool Whip Extra Creamy (nondairy), Dream Whip, and D-Zerta Whipped toppings all claim to be gluten-free.

Dessert Alert: Be suspicious of any ice cream product with cookies, brownies, cheesecake, or chips or candy mixed in. These can be ground so finely, you may not be aware of their presence. Be vigilant in frozen yogurts, especially in the new and very hot "fat-free" category.

TCBY and many other popular brands of the new nonfat frozen yogurts may contain malt and its chemical derivatives in order to flavor these "fabulous fakes." Watch out for Italian ices and sherbets too. Many contain modified food starch of an unspecified nature. Natural sorbets containing only fruit and added sugar are the better bet.

CEREALS AND CANDY

Kellogg's Corn Pops, General Mills' Cocoa Puffs, Malt-O-Meal Puffed Rice, Nabisco Cream of Rice, Post Fruity Pebbles, Quaker Puffed Rice and Quick Grits, and Ralston Purina Sun Flakes (corn and rice only) all claim to be gluten-free, but Kellogg's took the one I personally loved, Kennmei Rice Cereal, off the shelf. It's embarrassing for an adult to be caught eating Fruity Pebbles at a power breakfast!

Most corn or rice cereals contain malt flavoring, which is allowable for those on wheat-free diets, but not for those with celiac sprue. Malt must be avoided because it is purchased as a commodity by the food industry from the cheapest source. Because of that there is no control over whether it's corn malt (an okay kind) or barley malt (a no-no).

All licorice candy, red, black, and brown, contains wheat, and many jellied candies, such as gum drops and jelly beans, contain modified food starch and maltodextrin. Pure chocolate, such as Hershey's Kisses, plain or almond, are sweet revenge. If you think your favorite candy is gluten-free, call the manufacturer anyway.

Don't Forget! Many candies are passed along flour-coated conveyor belts in order to keep them from sticking during manufacture. Ask the maker of your favorite confection if wheat flour is used in the manufacturing process, and always let the customer service department know the seriousness of your reason for asking.

PASTA SAUCES

Newman's Own Sockarooni Spaghetti Sauce is gluten-free, as is Prego, Francesco Rinaldi, Classico d'Abruzzi, Ragu, and Con Agra's Healthy Choice. If you remember to read every label, in spite of the words *all natural* scrawled across the jar, you will do fine in this department.

MISCELLANEOUS

Musselman brand apple sauce, pie fillings, Dutch Baked Apples, and all other products from Lucky Leaf have been listed as gluten-free.

Kellogg's Corn Flake Crumbs are wheat-free, but contain malt and therefore are not gluten-free. General Foods' Shake 'n Bake barbecue recipe, chicken only, is gluten-free. Put on your sunglasses and roll right past pasta. Consider this an aerobic challenge—how many calories can *you* burn getting out of there?

Beware of exotic sauces, such as Hoisin sauce. It's full of flour. Forget duck sauce and those spicy black bean sauces, teriyaki glazes, stir-fry sauces, tamari and soy sauces. Buy only tamari and soy sauces that are clearly labeled wheat-free. Read oyster sauce labels carefully. Many are gluten-free, including a rather large selection of La Choy products from Beatrice/Hunt-Wesson.

Be wary of rice mixes, such as Rice-A-Roni, as any rice and sauce mix undoubtedly contains some form of dangerous grain.

Breyers yogurt is said to be made with all natural ingredients and therefore is gluten-free, but Dannon and Yoplait brands contain modified food starch.

Say no to Kraft Velveeta spread and Velveeta slices and Cheez Whiz and in fact, pass up anything that isn't simply cheese, plain and simple. Regular or whipped Philadelphia Cream Cheese is wheat- and gluten-free.

And remember what I said about those cooking oil sprays. Many contain grain alcohol. Cook with olive or canola oil. It's better for you.

CHECKOUT LINE

With pickings this slim, you should qualify for the express lane. If not, no nibbling while you wait. Buy Wrigley's gum and read about alien babies born to Hollywood stars instead.

It doesn't take a Ph.D. to see that you won't be spending too much quality time in the supermarket. Once you become familiar with what foods you can buy, the whole procedure should take about fifteen to thirty minutes. But before you decide to fill up the free hour with bowling lessons or Tai chi classes, you'd be advised to assess your alternative shopping skills.

The Health Food Store: What Is Your Tofu I.Q.?

If you think health food stores are the last refuge of tie-dye, mung bean sprouts, Birkenstock sandals, Zen macrobiotic behavior, plum balls, and hippies with stringy hair and neo-Bolshevik ideas, now is a good time to get over it. In other words, time saved in the supermarket would be better spent discovering your local health food establishment.

If you haven't yet noticed, health food has hit the mainstream. Holistic and herbal medicine and all manner of wheat, gluten-, egg-, dairy-, chemical-, pesticide-, and cruelty-free, organi-

AMARANTH. *Webster's* defines this ancient Aztec grain now enjoying new popularity among the health food cognoscenti as "from the Greek *amaranton* meaning unfading, a flower that never fades; any of a large genus of coarse herbs including pigweed (which is also known as tumbleweed in certain parts of the country) and various forms cultivated for their showy flowers or a dark reddish purple." Do not confuse amaranth with absinthe, which is rumored to be an aphrodisiac and is bad news for someone on the gluten-free diet. In its most common commercial form as a breakfast cereal, amaranth is loaded with oats, maltodextrin, and other ingredients that make this exotic a no-no.

cally pure, politically and environmentally correct, yin and yang, good-for-you products—Rice Dream frozen desserts, rice crust pizza, soy milk, wheat-free waffles, Mochi, almond milk, and organic take-out—are now being purchased and consumed with the frequency once reserved for the tuna casserole, and by nice, ordinary people who think amaranth (see page 40) is an aphrodisiac and Teff (see page 48) something that keeps food from sticking to the frying pan.

You will soon learn to love your local health food store, especially if you are lucky enough to live near one of those supermarket-slick emporiums once found only in California and in progressive university towns and that now seem to be popping up all over the country.

Having said this and having assumed you have gotten over all your silly, preestablished misconceptions regarding this "New Age" shopping experience, I suggest you grab the nearest straw, canvas, or string bag, jump into your Guatemalan huaraches, which are enjoying a real fashion comeback, and shop to your delicate little tummy's content.

If the products mentioned here are not available in your store, many company addresses and phone numbers are listed in chapter 12. Contact the company directly to arrange for shipping or to get the name of a distributor near you. Organic produce, prepared foods, and packaged products sold in health food stores cost more than supermarket products, but don't forget, due to the medical nature of your diet, you do have a tax advantage over other shoppers, which should take a little of the sting out of the total. Herewith, a walking tour of alternative shopping.

THE FREEZER CASE

The Original Rice Crust Pizza Company makes a rice-crust version of a frozen, pop-it-in-the-oven, supermarket pizza, complete with tomato and cheese topping. This comes in a soy cheese or an Italian cheese version. The crust tends to stick during cooking and I find spraying the cooking sheet with a little oil before baking eliminates the problem. Make sure your brand does not contain grain alcohol or, to be perfectly safe, use your own "spritz" bottle filled with olive oil.

The Organic Brown Rice Pizza Crust comes from Hilight (formerly Snack Cracks); you simply top it yourself and follow directions, again spraying the sheet before baking. The same company makes a Tostada "Pizza" that comes already topped with refried beans and cheese.

Waffles? Yes, waffles! Van's Wheat-Free, Gluten-Free Toaster Waffles are wonderful. Just add berries, jam, fresh fruit, gluten-free ice cream, or syrup.

Also in the freezer are Rudi's spelt bagels, hamburger buns, frozen bread sticks, plain spelt bread, and spelt raisin breads. Spelt (see the box on this page) has a nutty whole-grain taste that is tolerated by many people on wheat-free diets, but the product label on Rudi's products clearly states that you should check with your doctor before using them on a gluten-free diet. This is good advice for any "outsider grain" with which you are unfamiliar. Always read labels carefully.

> SPELT is a split piece of wood and the British past tense of the word *spell*. According to *Webster's New Collegiate Dictionary* it is also a form of wheat called Triticum spelta, with lax spikes and spikelets containing two light red kernels. Wheat by any other name is just as dangerous.
>
>

If you must have a hot dog and can't find a supermarket brand that does not contain cereal fillers and chemicals, or you're cutting down on animal protein, there are Soy Boy Not Dogs, one of the rare breeds of veggie dogs that does not list wheat or gluten as filler on the ingredient label. Warning: These are not for those of you with fond memories of the ball park. A ton of relish and gluten-free mustard is the trick to enjoying them fully.

Beware of Veggie Burgers! They almost always contain wheat and often contain seitan (see the box on page 48), the wheat gluten that gives them the texture and taste of meat.

Don't forget to stock up on yellow and blue corn tortillas, which, in addition to being gluten-free, are half the calories of their floury cousins. I steam them for eggs ranchero, substitute them for pita pockets, "rolled" sandwiches, enchiladas; bake them for quesadillas and Mexican pizza; fry them for homemade tortilla chips; float them in gazpacho; and always keep a supply in my freezer for bread emergencies.

For something faster, look in the freezer case for frozen enchiladas. Tumaro's frozen black bean enchiladas will do in a pinch.

The Refrigerator Case

In the refrigerator case you will find brown rice bread, yeast-free rice bread, and tapioca bread from Ener-G Foods, a mail-order company based in Seattle. It's always cheaper to buy than to ship, but if your health food store does not carry this brand or carries just a small selection, see chapter 4 for their full line of mail-order products. Do not attempt to eat this bread untoasted. Again, look very carefully at the labels on the various alternative breads and baked products displayed in this section. Some very exotic loaves, such as Kamut bread, (see the box on page 47 for more on kamut) not only contain gluten, but may contain more than wheat bread itself.

> **Warning:** Sprouted breads that are labeled "flourless" are not for you. It doesn't matter what form grain takes. You still can't digest it.

Baking Ingredients and Baked Goods

The baking aisle should yield quite an array of packaged flours. If you are lucky, your store carries Shiloh Farms wheat-, gluten-, and salt-free cake and cookie mixes, which can be substituted cup for cup for baking flour in any recipe.

One caveat: If your recipe calls for baking powder or baking soda, leave it out, it's already in these mixes. I didn't read the small print the first time I used the product, added the usual amount of baking powder, and Craig Claiborne's Christmas date nut loaf blew up in my oven. Days later my kitchen smelled like Windsor Castle after the Great

Fire. Always favoring the "slightly eccentric" solution, I managed to save the day by turning the unburned parts into a deep dish, topping it with a scoop of vanilla ice cream, calling it "crumble," and pretending I planned it that way.

If you are fortunate enough to live on the West Coast, you are likely to find Authentic Foods Bean Flour Baking Mixes, which are superb. If you don't, sources are listed in chapter 4.

David's Mr. Good Batter makes a wheat-free rice and oats pancake and baking mix and a wheat-free buttermilk pancake, waffle, and muffin mix, in addition to a gluten-free dark chocolate cake mix that makes the basis for a pretty decent old-fashioned iced cake when the mood strikes or when a birthday is imminent. Most health food stores carry gluten-free baking mixes from Ener-G Foods and Arrowhead Mills, among others.

Don't miss the cookie department, which, unlike the barren shelves of its supermarket counterpart, is full of sweet revenge and more than a few extra pounds of pure butter. Pamela's Products makes a dense, blissfully gluten-free cocoa shortbread cookie, chunky chocolate chip, and wheat-free oatmeal date coconut and oatmeal raisin walnut varieties. Also in the wheat-, but not gluten-free category, chocolate chocolate chunk and date almond cookies from Lady J. and three types from Nature's Warehouse—chocolate, chocolate chip with walnuts, and walnut multi-grain, also wheat-free only. Gold Mine makes wheat-free fig bars and apple cinnamon fig bars, as well as wheat-free cookies in devil's food and caramel crisp. Mr. Densen's

SOME QUESTIONS: Have you noticed that, in the health food store, products you can eat are clearly labeled wheat- or gluten-free, while in the supermarket they are not? Have you wondered why this is? Could it be that some companies care about their customers' health and others do not? Shouldn't all labels declare the contents thus? Why not write to your government representative and pose these questions?

makes a wheat-free oatmeal raisin cookie and a wheat-free vanilla chip macaroon.

In the oversize, individually wrapped category, Healthy Munchies makes a yeast-free, wheat-free cookie, as does the Integrity Baking Company; its brand is Wheatless Maple Walnut Cookie. Glenny's Brown Rice Treat sounds gluten-free, but it contains barley malt. Fran's Fresh Foods makes an all-natural, individually wrapped, preservative- and wheat-free cherry cobbler muffin; Abraham's Natural Foods makes a similar "free" jumbo sweet rice cookie. Write for a complete wheat- and gluten-free selection of products.

PASTA

If there is any room left in your shopping cart, head for the pasta aisle and weep for joy.

My hands-down favorite is Pastariso, a nutty and delicious, blissfully gluten-free, brown rice pasta that comes in a red, white, and green box and takes the form of fettuccine, spaghetti, fusilli, elbows, and rice twists. This is the pasta I serve to my favorite people with a beautiful pesto made from garden-grown basil or with fresh tomato sauce and watch them beg for the recipe, which I always give. Even better, it's half the calories of semolina. Who says there is no justice in the world?

Another respectable gluten-free pasta comes from Ener-G Foods and takes the form of vermicelli, shells, spaghetti, and cannelloni. My personal favorite is their lasagne noodle, which, when layered, sauced, and cheesed up, is just as satisfying as the real thing, as long as you cook the noodle al dente. (It will cook a bit more while baking.)

In the wheat- but not gluten-free category, Vita Spelt makes lasagne, angel hair, shells, rotini, spaghetti, and a premixed macaroni and cheese dinner.

Ancient Quinoa Harvest, I am told, makes an interesting and nutty-tasting wheat-free pasta in elbows, shells, rotelle, and multicolor shapes called Garden Pagoda that would look great against a nice green pesto. (The box says gluten-free, the Celiac Disease Foundation says yes, *The Merck Manual* says no, and so do the people at the Celiac Sprue Association/USA. Personally, I'm afraid to try it. I'd get a medical opinion before buying this controversial grain.)

DeBoles Nutritional Foods makes elbows and spaghetti it describes as "imitation corn pasta" (the last time I looked, yellow cornmeal and yellow corn flour *were* real foods) and is advertised as wheatfree, but based on the ingredients, appears to be gluten-free as well. Many of this company's products contain semolina, so read package labels very carefully. However inappropriate its usage, the word *imitation* is the tip-off to the one you can eat.

QUINOA, pronounced keen-wa, is Inca for "the mother grain." According to the legend on the back of the box, it was so crucial to the Inca diet that the king planted the first row of quinoa each season with a solid gold spade. Ancient affluence aside, quinoa dates back over five thousand years. This tiny kernel that is no bigger than a mustard seed once fed an entire civilization. Maybe it was sprue, not the Spanish, that caused the Incas to disappear. Do not allow it to cause you to disappear. Is it gluten-free? There are many opinions. Get your doctor's.

While you are in the market for carbohydrates, don't miss the Asian section for rice noodles called bi-fun, bean thread, and cellophane. Pure buckwheat noodles, or udon, as the Japanese call them, are virtually impossible to find, and most brands are mixed with semolina. Worse, the labels are in Japanese.

BUCKWHEAT is not a member of the wheat family at all. It's a fruit, really, and comes closer to the density of animal protein than any other plant. Despite its unfortunate name and the fact that it is on the Merck list of no-nos, some say buckwheat is gluten-free. If you like this heavy stuff, get a third opinion.

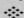

JAPANESE PRODUCTS

The Japanese shelf should also yield a more interesting array of wheat-free and, therefore, gluten-free, soy and tamari sauces, brown rice, and plum vinegars than your supermarket.

Look for entries from Eden, Tree of Life, Mitoku Macrobiotic, Ohsawa, and Westbrae Natural Foods. Read all wheat-free sauce and vinegar labels for the presence of barley before deciding the product is also gluten-free.

Always watch for products that contain soy sauce. You never know whether it is regular or wheat-free.

CEREAL

Interest heats up in hot cereals. Lundberg Family Farms makes a hearty and delicious rice cereal in almond date, cinnamon raisin, and

TEMPEH is not a place in Arizona. It is a low-fat source of protein made from soybeans and can be sautéed, steamed, baked, barbecued, used as a bread substitute in meatballs, or diced and simmered in soups and stews. It is gluten-free as long as it is sold in its natural state (faintly gray and packed in squares) and not used as an ingredient or mixed with soy sauce made from fermented wheat.

KAMUT, pronounced ka-moot, is an ancient Peruvian member of the wheat family that is very low in gluten and often can be tolerated by those who are allergic to wheat. Check with your doctor before trying this and never eat kamut on a gluten-free diet.

original flavors. Rice and Shine is the smoothie from Arrowhead Mills, and American Quinoa Harvest makes a hot and satisfying wheat-free bowl of quinoa flakes, among others.

In the stick-to-your-ribs department, nothing beats Pocono Heart of Buckwheat roasted buckwheat groats (kasha), if your doctor permits it. According to the box, the real secret to a light, fluffy texture is to seal kasha kernels with an egg before pouring on hot liquid. Write for the company's cookbook.

Watch for barley malt in the cold cereals. That is what disqualifies most supermarket brands and it's what will keep you from health food store flakes as well. Most are wheat-free but not gluten-free. Erewhon corn flakes are the exception. Learn to spot the difference.

> SEITAN is high-density wheat gluten used by vegetarians to make fake meat. Avoid it at all costs.
>
>

BEVERAGES

For those of you who are thirsty, don't care for the chemicals in most soft drinks, and may have a touch of lactose intolerance, Vitasoy makes refreshing lactose-free soy milks in such flavors as cocoa, vanilla, carob, and Creamy Original.

> TEFF is not a nonstick coating for cookware. It is the smallest grain in the world and has, for thousands of years, been the grain of choice for the baking of injera, a traditional Ethiopian flat bread. It is wheat- but not gluten-free.
>
>

ICE CREAM

If you scream for ice cream and feel strongly about saving the sea turtles, you are in for a treat. Sweet Nothings is a line of all-natural, nondairy frozen desserts from Turtle Mountain, Inc. Like our friends Ben & Jerry, who also work for good causes, 1 percent of their profits goes toward the future of these lovable slowpokes. Call first, then enjoy the stuff in endangered flavors such as Tiger Stripes (vanilla and fudge), Black Leopard (chocolate, coffee, and cinnamon), and other exotics such as Espresso Fudge, Very Berry Blueberry, Mango Raspberry, and Raspberry Swirl. For the full-fat dairy variety of frozen dessert, look for Stars, a line of desserts from the same company.

CARRAGEEN GUM is derived from a dark-purple, cartilaginous seaweed commonly called Irish moss that is found on the coasts of northern Europe and America. It is used most often as a suspension agent in frozen confections. It is a safe additive.

Other brands that do not list wheat or gluten on their labels (always check with the company!) and can satisfy the craving for ice cream and frozen yogurt are Rice Dream nondairy dessert (good for lactose intolerance too); Stonyfield Farm nonfat frozen yogurt in divine flavors such as mocha fudge, walnut amaretto, and almond fudge; Cascadian Farm frozen yogurts and yogurt bars; Ice Bean Organic Frozen Dessert; and an all-natural ice cream from Alta Dena Certified Dairy, each container of which bears a plant identification number for questions and reference. Check all frozen dessert labels for fillers and other hidden glutens and remember, ingredients always vary from flavor to flavor.

DRESSINGS, SAUCES, AND SOUPS

If you crave a change from Newman's Own dressings, investigate Anne's Original 1850 Farmhouse Salad Dressings, but pass up her Big Martin's Dijon & Horseradish Vinaigrette, which contains mustard, and Uncle Chang's Sesame Seed flavor, which contains soy sauce. Also look for Blanchard and Blanchard low-fat Spa Dressings. As with everything, write or call these companies for the last word.

Always be on guard for soy sauce, tamari, mustard, and white vinegar in health food store dressings, and hold the mayo. The "natural" brands tend to contain grain vinegar and, truthfully, Hellman's is about as good as it gets. Tree of Life organic mustard and Hain's natural stone-ground mustard both contain cider vinegar, which makes them gluten-free. Ditto for Enrico's Ketchup and Uncle Dave's. Both list cider vinegar instead of white vinegar.

Always read pasta sauce labels carefully, even though they advertise all-natural ingredients prominently. Enrico's, Uncle Dave's, Millena's Finest, and Muir Glen Organic Pasta Sauces are among my favorites.

The soup shelf here is a much more comforting place than the supermarket's. Hain's Chicken Broth, Vegetable Chicken, Minestrone, Vegetarian Split Pea, Vegetarian Vegetable Broth, Vegetarian Lentil, Black Bean and Wild Rice as well as Health Valley fat-free 14 Garden Vegetable, 5 Bean Vegetable, Lentil & Carrots, Tomato Vegetable, Country Corn & Vegetable, Split Pea & Carrots, and Black Bean & Vegetables list no wheat or gluten on their labels. I find many of these soups bland, and you may want to "doctor" them with your own seasonings as I do. Pass up Pritikin soups. Most contain food starch and wheat flour.

SNACKS

Unlike the mainstream market, there's plenty of good, gluten-free snacking in crackers, rice cakes, and snacks. If you are tired of the same old snacks, Terra Chips in sweet potato or mixed exotic vegetables make a welcome change from corn and rice. Barbara's Pinta Chips are a tangy salsa combination of salsa and pinto beans. Both brands claim to be wheat- and gluten-free. Edward & Sons makes Brown Rice Snaps and uses wheat-free tamari in the recipe. Hain's makes many Mini Popcorn Cakes in many varieties. Mothers products are widely represented here, and one of my personal favorites is Tree of Life fat-free, bite-size caramel rice cakes. All of these appear to be

gluten-free as do many others in this section. Watch out for flavors
that may contain wheat-based soy sauce or tamari.

> WHEY. According to *Webster's New Collegiate Dictionary*, this is
> "the serum or watery part of milk that is separated from the co-
> agulable part or curd esp. in the process of making cheese and
> that is rich in lactose, minerals, and vitamins and contains lactal-
> bumin and traces of fat." In other words, unless you are lactose
> intolerant, there's no need to stay away from whey.
>
>

THE DAIRY CASE

Stonyfield Farm makes a great-tasting and very creamy acidopho-
lous culture yogurt with no artificial sweeteners, both in nonfat and
regular varieties. Also, if you suffer problems with lactose, there are
many "cheeses" here for you.

Okay. You're really into this alternative shopping thing, "feeling your
oats," so to speak.

Buy yourself some mochi (pronounced moe-chee). These individually wrapped rice goodies may look and feel like floor tiles, but once
you slice them along their prescored lines and bake, they puff up into
crunchy-on-the-outside, sticky-in-the-middle little muffins in pizza
flavor, raisin and cinnamon, and plain rice. Avoid sesame garlic (it contains soy sauce) and mugwort (it contains wheat grass).

While you're at it, fry up some tempeh for sandwiches, burritos,
or fajitas. It comes in Corn Jalapeño and Garden Vegetable varieties
from Light Life Foods.

Don't miss masa or masa harina—no, it's not the hill with a flat
top—it's the centuries'-old corn mixture from 21st Century Foods, as
well as hummus (a chickpea paste flavored with tahini sauce and garlic), stuffed grape leaves, daikon pickles, Amazaki sweet rice shakes,

baba ghanouj and of course, tofu. Tofu, an unattractive, jiggly soy bean curd, is really one of the all-time wonder foods. It is extremely high in protein, gluten-free, and, because it has virtually no taste of its own, it is a true chameleon, taking on any flavor you give it. It can be fried, steamed, grilled, broiled, baked, mashed, diced, pureed to make creamy desserts, and substituted for any other food. Tofu is more than a food in Japan. It is a ritual. We'll save it for next time: Marketing 102.

CHAPTER THREE

Attitude. Attitude. Attitude.

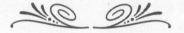

I got a new attitude . . .
—PATTY LaBELLE

Any streetwise, inner-city kid will tell you, survival is 10 percent smarts and 90 percent attitude. With three squares, two snacks, and a midnight nibble at stake every day for the rest of your life, you're going to have to do a lot more than survive.

While it's true you may have enough wheat- and gluten-free food stashed in your kitchen to last through the millennium, you can't stay home and munch rice crackers forever. Sooner or later you must sit down to a meal with other humans. How well you do is going to depend heavily on your attitude.

Is the stomach half full or half empty? Is the patient half sick or half well? Do you see two perfectly poached eggs slathered in silky Hollandaise beckoning to you from matching slabs of honey-baked ham? Or do you merely see the English muffin?

Your answers to these and other important questions will determine how hard it's going to be for you to make your way in a world that is much more comfortable saying no than yes; that would have you suffer in silence rather than give you special treatment; and that would have you believe being different is tantamount to being sick.

The attitudinal trick is to see yourself as perfectly healthy or, to be more precise, no longer sick, in spite of the fact that your plumbing is peculiar at best, your immune system is so weird it sees an innocent chunk of bread as a deadly poison, and your genetic structure probably should be displayed in Ripley's Believe It or Not.

The problem is, other people always confuse healthy, which you are now or soon will be, with normal, which you are decidedly not. Anyone who can't eat pizza, chocolate chip cookies, apple pie, hot dogs, hush puppies, and hamburgers is not only considered abnormal, in certain small towns and villages the unfortunate may even be considered a threat to society. To decline the foods so symbolic of our culture's preoccupation with Mom, the flag, instant gratification, and empty calories is to be met with narrow-eyed suspicion at best.

My advice is to stop trying to pass yourself off as normal. To be accurate as well as politically correct, you are "nutritionally challenged." The sooner you digest this important distinction, the sooner you can stop seeing your diet as an obstacle to pleasure and start approaching it in a way that allows for maximum possibility. The goal is not simply eating, it's eating well; not merely getting a meal on the table, but getting a great one on the table. If this is to be achieved with any regularity, the solution must be as unusual as the problem. It's really as simple as that. The harder you try to fit in, the hungrier you get. Look at it another way: Your body has been eccentric for years, why shouldn't you?

The night I slipped a demitasse spoon out of my evening bag and headed for the caviar was the first time I realized this. If I had insisted on seeing myself as normal, I would have behaved in a way that was appropriate to the situation. I might have spooned some caviar onto a cracker and tried discreetly to scrape off a bit of roe with my teeth, risking a potentially nasty spill, which is not a great idea in a new evening dress, or worse, I might have not tried at all and begun the New Year with a great big helping of self-pity.

By seeing myself not as unwell but as rare and unusual and, by virtue of my peculiar and special genetic makeup, one who is allowed to break the rules, I was able to enjoy my fill of one of my favorite foods. In the process, I began the necessary shift in attitude that brings with it self-respect, self-reliance, a sense of adventure, a sense of being in control, and more than its share of good things to eat. By giving myself permission to be creative about my problem, I was able to apply the principle of old-fashioned positive thinking and come up with an elegant solution that fit the festive tone of the evening.

It tickles me today to know that the other guests did not see my odd eating style for what it really was—a clever way around a tough problem—and I smile when I see that others, thinking I am a connoisseur, have on successive evenings copied my behavior, waving their spoons and proclaiming their passion for the stuff. Last year I actually overheard a gentleman who witnessed my now-annual descent-into-caviar-with-spoon dismissing the cracker, as well as the chopped egg and onion, as "irrelevant to the enjoyment of good Sevruga."

I admit this behavior may seem a bit crazy by some standards, especially to those poor lemmings who sleep-walk through life with a rule book bolted to their heads, but think of the alternative—a howling empty place in your stomach and in your soul that gets bigger and bigger with every meal. Does it really matter what others think?

If carrying your own spoon to cocktail parties isn't comfortable for you at first, start small. Carry two slices of rice bread to a restaurant, ask the waiter to toast it, then order any sandwich on the menu. Ditto for dipping, mopping, sopping, burgers, grilled cheese, tuna melts, Reubens, and ordering eggs Benedict, once you have thoroughly investigated the hollandaise, of course.

Forget plastic baggies. These will turn your bread into instant bread crumbs. Measure your favorite loaf and find yourself an attractive plastic container that holds two slices securely. Prowl the flea markets, pick up a campy child's lunch box from the fifties, and use that to keep your bread and crackers fresh. Trust me, people will copy your style, especially if you're lucky enough to find a vintage Hopalong Cassidy or Betty Boop or Yosemite Sam. Why not have one made to measure in silver or wood? You're going to use it often, so why not splurge on something that looks great? (You had nice lighters when you smoked, didn't you?) Just make sure the waiter returns it. Some years ago I found a lovely old miniature silver hinged box of the type Victorian women dangled from their belts and their bosoms. They filled them with mysterious things—lace hankies, a lock of their lover's hair, some snuff, that teensy vial of laudanum I imagine gave them the dreamy look they always seemed to wear. I slip mine on a velvet ribbon and wear it to parties. People are amazed to find such a lovely object home to my personal cache of rice crackers.

For those occasions that warrant gooey cheeses, finger foods, and lots of dips, carry a bag full of rice crackers and make sure you wear something with deep pockets. Slip them out one at time (or ask for your own small serving bowl) and nosh to your heart's content. And don't try to hide what you're doing. This is a great conversation starter as long as you don't belabor it and, God forbid, get trapped in a discussion of the medical reasons for your unusual social behavior.

For longer eating experiences, such as weekends at the beach or family visits, fill a bag with your own food. This may sound awfully self-centered, but it is really quite thoughtful, both for you and your host, who is responsible not only for your comfort and pleasure but for every guest's comfort and pleasure for the duration.

If I have to travel for business for an extended period of time, I ship a carton of my goodies to myself, care of the hotel, then alert the chef and the room service manager to my special needs. It's amazing what two slices of rice toast or a wheat- and gluten-free muffin served on a tray can do for your spirits and your stress level when you are working away from home.

The idea is to do whatever it takes to help you feel as special as you are in every way possible and to put the power back where it belongs—with you, not with your diet. With apologies to John Fitzgerald Kennedy, "Yours is not to ask why, but to ask why not." Naturally, your new and more confident self will not appear overnight, but if you follow these steps, you too will be packing small spoons, asking for sliced cucumbers, waving your bread at waiters, and demanding (always politely) that your special foods be presented to you on a silver platter. Carried off properly, the right attitude celebrates your uniqueness and can, with the appropriate tilt of the nose and a well-timed lift of an eyebrow, even offer a touch of sympathy for those unlucky enough to be ordinary.

Before you can move ahead, however, you must go back—all the way back to the beginning—and adjust. How tough an adjustment this is really depends on who you are; how much self-esteem and con-

fidence you possess; how much self-examination you've been exposed
to; where you are, high to low, on the risk-aversion scale; how seriously you take yourself and your dietary circumstances; and how willing you are to appear foolish to strangers.

The important thing to know is that it is absolutely within your
power to change in a more positive way, to become more resourceful
about your diet and more forthright in presenting it to others. No
major personal overhaul is required here, nor is the prerequisite thirty
years of painful therapy. Just some minor revisions in the way you look
at life in general and your diet problems specifically, and you may find
you're a whole lot healthier than you ever imagined.

Attitude Adjustment No. 1
First you mourn.

It is so easy to feel guilty about grieving for something the rest of
the world perceives as unimportant. After all, people are dying and all
you have is a little problem with grain. Right? Wrong.

If you haven't moaned and complained, kicked and screamed,
whimpered, whined "Why me?" and refused to be in the same room
with spaghetti, you must do so now. Without the sadness and the
anger and the acknowledgment of how serious this problem is for you,
that it will be with you for the rest of your life, there *is* no new attitude.
There is only the downward spiral of self-pity and denial, guilt and
self-destructive behavior that leads to the never-ending cycle of more
of the same. To use food terms, if you don't allow yourself to grieve
openly, your resentment will simmer and boil over, eventually scalding
everyone in its path. Wallow away.

Attitude Adjustment No. 2
Accept that you are powerless over your diet.

Beyond pain is acceptance and beyond that is recovery. I'm not
talking about recovery in the look-Ma-I-can-eat-grain-again sense. I'm
talking about recovering your balance, your good humor, your ability
to see yourself not as ill but as a creative person who uses his or her

natural resourcefulness to enjoy life and to maintain health, someone who can say "it's no big deal" and mean it. To borrow a bit of wisdom from Alcoholics Anonymous's Twelve Step program, you can't develop a healthy attitude toward your food intolerance until you admit that you are powerless over it.

Like everyone who has ever had to face a disability—and yes, this is a disability just like any other—the sooner you accept the unalterable fact of it, the sooner you can move beyond it to the strategy for coping with it creatively and positively.

Put another way, the energy it takes to deny the problem, ignore it, trivialize it, pretend it's not there, wish it weren't, and suppress your true feelings about it can now be used to a better purpose.

Attitude Adjustment No. 3
Complain. Explain.

We don't ask a person who is trying to quit smoking to empty the ashtrays; nor do we send a drinking problem to the liquor store for a nice California Chardonnay. So why do we ask people on restrictive diets to prepare our meals?

I've seen this happen to people, usually women, who are trying to lose weight, eating almost nothing while continuing to prepare enormous, high-calorie meals for their families. The dieter weighs in with radishes and cottage cheese while the rest of the family eat like longshoremen after a hard day on the docks. The same is true for those of us who must follow a grain-restricted diet. This is even more unfair because our problems will not melt away like so many extra pounds, a temporary inconvenience until the goal is reached.

At my house, no one would dream of asking me to toast an English muffin; not because my husband guessed that I can't bear that singular aroma and the way butter disappears into all the little nooks and crannies, but because I told him how hard it is for me, how sad I feel when I do it. Waiting for people magically to understand your needs is always unrealistic; expecting a spouse or children or good friends to know at any given moment which food cues upset you is asking for trouble.

I am reminded of the neighbor who is working up the courage to ask his neighbor if he can borrow a ladder. He thinks about the chances of his neighbor lending it to him with generosity and thinks, "Well, after all, I loaned him my electric drill." A little while later he remembers the time the neighbor took a month to return a barbecue fork. And even later in the day, still worrying about whether his request will be met with a negative response, it occurs to him that his auto buffing attachment has never been returned. Finally, several hours later, the man marches across his neighbor's lawn, rings the doorbell, and when the unsuspecting man answers, he shouts, "You know something, I don't want your damn ladder anyway!" and stomps off.

It's tempting to find fault with the people who ask us to cook for them. After all, that's selfish, isn't it? Not really. The blame lies not with those who expect us to continue making dinner, but with the one who doesn't protest this unfair arrangement. A gluten-free diet is bad enough; suffering in silence is stupid.

Attitude Adjustment No. 4
Communicate. Negotiate.

Sighing, rolling eyes, and looks of martyred despair went out with Melanie and Ashley, *Little Women,* and *My Little Margie.* Speak up. Tell all the people who love you how hard it is for you to watch them butter a piece of bread.

Old patterns must change and family traditions need to be adjusted if you are to succeed and your diet is to be acknowledged, not as an afterthought but in a meaningful way. While everyone must understand how serious and important the elimination of wheat and gluten from your diet really is for you, it is your responsibility to tell them, not theirs to guess.

As with everything in life, no one is going to respond to your needs unless you tell them what those needs are. If you don't, believe me, you will find ways to make them pay for their lack of clairvoyance. The important thing is not to pile one resentment on top of the other in a kind of *pousse café* of grievances until no one remembers, least of all you, how many layers of anger make up this lethal and destructive cocktail, but to get those feelings out in the open, theirs as well as yours, as they occur. Here are some ways to get off to a good start.

1. If you are the primary chef in the family, you may want to let go of this responsibility for a while and explain that preparing "normal" food is hard for you. In fact, you may find one meal more difficult to prepare for others than another. Breakfast, for example, is the most brutal for me because I really miss bagels and croissants and all those crunchy granola cereals that are the backbones of this grain-based meal. Tell your family exactly how you feel when you watch them munch toast. (I unconsciously chew along with people, like a passenger who brakes from the backseat!)

2. Hold a family meeting to discuss food preparation options and develop a rotating schedule, so no one is ever stuck with fixing the same meal for longer than a week. Include everyone in the family, even the youngest members, so everyone plays a part. Review the schedule weekly or monthly as your own feelings change.

3. Elicit your family's feelings about your not wanting to prepare certain foods for them any longer. Discuss your sadness or feelings of deprivation when faced with specific food situations, such as family picnics, pizza night, mall food, preparing sandwiches for school lunches, special occasions. Talk about birthdays and holidays, and ask them to think of ways to make them easier on you.

Believe it or not, one birthday I was surprised with a cake by well-meaning coworkers who actually thought it would please me to blow out the candles, then watch them devour it. Another year a relative prepared the family Thanksgiving dinner without a single dish I could eat. People need to know how disappointing and upsetting those occasions are for you.

4. If there is one food in particular, such as brownies or chocolate chip cookies or marble pound cake or brioche, that you can't stand to see being enjoyed, ask family, friends, and receptive coworkers that it not be eaten in your presence.

5. Tell family members ahead of time that you will not be preparing meals for multiple diets. Be very clear in letting them know whatever is good for you will have to be good for them and ask for their understanding about this. Find out what their gluten-free favorites are and be as inventive with their meals as you are with yours.

The more people who enjoy your food, the less isolated you'll feel, so make a game of it. My husband has developed a real preference for rice now that I have learned to do so much with it, and his reaction when I prepare risotto or jambalaya can hardly be characterized as disappointment. Glee is more like it when I offer grilled polenta with a savory sun-dried tomato and mushroom sauce and freshly grated Parmesan. Who says selfishness isn't kind?

6. Communication works both ways. Listen carefully to how other people feel about this change in their lives and try to be just as understanding and accommodating when loved ones express sadness or anger at their own loss as a result of your diet. Try to understand.

This is easy to intellectualize, but when your family tells you they're all going out for pizza and have not invited you so they can enjoy it without having to bear the guilt of gobbling it up in your presence, it's hard to be gracious and easy to feel sorry for yourself. You'll get better at this with time. Try to thank them for their consideration, even if you don't feel particularly grateful yet. A healthy attitude doesn't mean life is a one-way street in your direction. It means being sensitive to the needs of others as well as to your own, even if it hurts, and it does.

7. Be open. Be willing to compromise, such as by saying, "I'll make lunch, if you take care of your own breakfast." Remember, children have very strong feelings about being cared for and nurtured, and they really can't understand a parent's problem unless they are directly told. Consider this talk with your child as a lesson in becoming an adult who isn't afraid to ask for special attention. If you honor your children with their own importance in your life, they will honor you. They will also grow up honoring themselves. Never underestimate them.

When you are comfortable that your family understands this important change in your life, broaden the communication to friends, relatives, and co-workers, people with whom you are not necessarily intimate but who may be in a position to cook or order food for you, such as a secretary, company steward, cafeteria manager, corporate meeting planner. Here it is important to state the problem and what you require of people without baring as much of yourself as you have to your immediate family and closest friends. (Hint: Your office rival is not the one with whom to discuss your deep sense of loss over cheese Danish.)

A word of warning here—controlling someone's food is as close to controlling the person as it gets. Be prepared for some disappointments, even some nasty surprises. There will be people who will always find a reason to forget your special diet and who never seem to have extra goodies on hand for you. Asking people to extend themselves may unearth some negative feelings toward you, ones that may have lain dormant until now.

If there are unresolved issues or negative feelings between you and the people you are asking to help you, it may be impossible for them to extend themselves until those issues are brought out in the open. Be direct. Ask why they never remember your problem. You may be surprised at the answer.

For some, the extra effort just may be impossible because what you're really asking them to do is change their behavior, and many people simply can't or won't do that. Others can't accept it when someone in their circle changes, voluntarily or not.

I've seen this happen in very serious instances where a friend is faced with a sudden change in economic status, a severe physical impairment, and even the tragedy of diminished mental capacity. It has happened to me. In each instance the person has asked for support in accordance with the circumstances, and it may as well have never been said. Everyone listens, but some never hear. You too will expect the best and, sadly, discover the basic selfishness and inflexibility of some. In some cases, the awakening will be rude and, in others, a blessing you never knew you had, but I think in the end, if you'll pardon the expression, the wheat will separate from the chaff.

Attitude Adjustment No. 5
Never trivialize your problem or allow others to do so.

The word *just* no longer exists for you. Never use this sloppy little adverb to present your problem to the world. I'm referring to the popular usage, "Oh, it's just a little grain problem" or "It's just an allergy." When you speak this way, you are belittling the importance of your problem, and it is a cue for others to do the same.

People who deliberately minimize the importance of their diets remind me of the old joke that asks, How many martyrs does it take to change a light bulb?

None. They'd rather sit in the dark.

Words such as *just, only,* and *merely* fly in the face of all that you are. Whenever you use them, you are begging the listener to turn off and not to take you or your request seriously. Habits like this are tough to break because something in your background is telling you you don't deserve the full attention of others, that your problems are not as important as theirs. Short of years of expensive therapy, the following affirmation can help you see yourself differently. (An affirmation is something you say or write over and over until you begin to believe it.)

"I, _____, am a unique and special person worthy of all the special attention, love, and understanding I ask from those around me."

Fill in your name and write this affirmation in a small notebook or on an index card you can carry with you at all times. When you feel that you are about to trivialize your needs or reject special attention from people, take it out and remind yourself that you deserve only the best from yourself and from other people.

Developing a new attitude means developing a new response to old cues. People will tell you how lucky you are that it's "just" (there's that word again) a diet and nothing worse. Depending on your relationship, there are many ways to deal with this, none of which includes agreement because agreeing with someone else's judgment about how you should feel is tantamount to being rendered invisible and invalid.

Over time you will develop your own responses that will suit the situation and your relationship to the person who has spoken carelessly or behaved in a way you find unacceptable, disappointing, or intolerable. For now, here are some stock answers that will let others know you are not a person to be dismissed and will leave you feeling a whole lot better for having stood up for yourself. If someone is rude and/or dumb enough to say, "You know, you really should feel lucky it's just an allergy and not something worse," match the punishment with the crime:

a. "Maybe I will at some point, but right now this is really tough for me."
b. "I'll let you know when I do."
c. "Why don't you try my diet for a week, then tell me how lucky you feel."
d. "Do me a favor, don't visit someone who's just had a mastectomy, okay?"

You will find yourself in food situations where someone in your family or circle of friends has forgotten you completely. As sure as the sun comes up, they will try to cover their embarrassment by saying something stupid and insensitive. Naturally, you must gauge your response to the intention and measure it according to how often you have been offended by this person.

My own experience is that most people usually forget once. After a gentle reminder, they more than make it up to you the next time. One or two may forget so often, you have no recourse but to question their motives, decline their invitations, and examine the shaky ground on which your relationship is built. The subtlety or vehemence of your response naturally will depend on whether food is central to the occasion—you're not going to tell the recently bereaved at the funeral luncheon that she forgot your rice bread, no matter how close the two of you are. Let the punishment fit the criminal as well as the crime. Sooner or later, someone is bound to say, "Oh, I forgot. You can't eat that." You say:

a. "It's my fault. I really should have phoned ahead to remind you."
b. "If making special food is a problem for you, let me know and I'll bring my own food next time."
c. "Tell you what, next time you invite me, I'll forget to come."

Another common stupid comment is the one usually delivered by your brother-in-law Boomer or your Aunt Martha after he or she realizes you've just been served a slice of flourless chocolate cake (safe) with a cookie crust (not safe). Instead of apologizing profusely and getting you some fruit, the guilty party compounds the insult by acknowledging the error in a way that gets him or her off the hook and you squarely on it. This little face-saving, guest-embarrassing tactic is a question you will hear much too often: "Why don't you just eat the middle?"

It's tough to remain unruffled, hang on to your dignity, and be firm in your resolve never to reduce yourself to doing any such thing in the face of such an obvious deflective maneuver, but it is possible with any one of these.

a. "No, thanks. I'd really rather not risk getting something that might make me ill."
b. "No, thanks. I don't really enjoy picking my food apart."
c. "Great idea. Why don't we all eat the middles!"

Of course, if you're really disgusted, have heard this too often, and have given serious thought to the wisdom of accepting any further invitations from this particular person, you do have other options.

a. "Why don't you eat the middle too and let me know how *you* like it?"
b. "Clearly you enjoy watching me suffer."
c. "Why don't you just put my dish on the floor with the dog's?"

Attitude Adjustment No. 6
Pity is not positive.

Reject negative attention politely and firmly. All that poor-you stuff does not contribute to a good attitude, nor does it inspire creativity.

Slowly and insidiously, the pity of others can erode self-esteem and may even contribute to a victim mentality. You may find yourself always presenting that needy side of yourself to the person who constantly encourages it, and it also may result in your being viewed as a victim and less than equal in other areas of the relationship.

It's easy to fall into this trap, especially just after diagnosis when you are feeling sorry for yourself, but beware of the person who does not encourage you to get over it, who whispers to others about how hard it is for you to live on this diet, who is always there to pat your hand and remind you how badly you feel about pasta, and who, in so many insidious ways disguised as concern, keeps you in that swamp so long, you forget all the other things you are, seeing yourself only as the one who can't eat wheat and other grains. That's a pretty narrow view of yourself. You really don't need people who work hard to make sure that's the only one you see.

Naturally, you must learn to distinguish between an unhealthy focus on your problems and real compassion and caring. The fastest way to do this is to see what action follows. People who use pity to keep the people in their lives feeling as badly as they no doubt do often don't follow through with positive action; true compassion and healthy caring usually result in wonderful surprises, special foods, generous ideas, pantries permanently stocked with goodies for you, and very little talk about your diet beyond learning more about how to make it easier and more pleasant for you.

We pay dearly for being coddled. You simply have to be willing to give it up. You don't need it or the people who indulge your need for it. But you know that.

Attitude Adjustment No. 7
The harder you work, the better you eat.

From here on in, you have to participate in the process. Every meal in. Every breakfast, lunch, and dinner out. Every bite on the road, at the mall, in a plane, at the park. Every time. And it's work.

When we visit friends, we can't just hand them a list of what foods we must avoid. We have to teach them how to make the foods we can eat. We have to make sure they're using the right mayonnaise or mustard; that their corn bread is all corn; that their barbecue sauce contains no white vinegar, their marinade is not soy. If necessary, we must supply these things.

Nor can we afford to turn up our noses at the precious few prepared foods available to us, because we can't simply switch brands like everybody else. We have to learn how to doctor them—add extra chocolate and nuts, a layer of raspberry jam or a decadent icing to wheat- and gluten-free cake and brownie mixes; slice fresh fruit into muffin recipes, or reinvent breakfast cereals with extra raisins, bits of dried fruit, and shredded coconut. If we want cheesecake or pie, we can't simply order or bake them, we have to guide the cook in adapting their recipes for us or figure out which gluten-free cookie (my two favorites are ginger and cocoa) to substitute for the normal crust or topping and do it ourselves. Often we are forced to prepare an entire dessert just because we crave one serving. If we don't trust ourselves to deposit the remainder in the freezer or if the recipe doesn't keep, we find ourselves hosting more than our share of dinner parties.

We have to know the ingredients in foods sold by vendors of every description well before we are struck with the urge to buy ourselves an ice cream cone, French fries, or a banana smoothie. We have to be willing to prepare the meal, host the party, do dessert, bring a casserole, roast the turkey, and make the stuffing in order to be sure we're going to enjoy it. If we're not, we will be disappointed. Guaranteed.

The adjustment to this new "interactive" eating can be daunting, but you have to realize the world cooks and eats a certain way and it's not going to change for you.

The bottom line—you can no longer sit back and be served, and the desire to give up and eat something out of a can or a frozen food tray will be very strong at times.

Attitude Adjustment No. 8
Assume nothing and never take yes for an answer.

Periodically, phone, write, and fax any company that makes a wheat- and gluten-free product you happen to like. Just because it was wheat- or gluten-free when you read the label doesn't mean it will always remain so. Many food marketers buy their ingredients from different suppliers, and changes are not reflected on labels that must be printed well in advance. You don't have to be paranoid, but you do have to be careful.

The operative attitude is "I'm the customer and you are in business to please me and to make sure I don't get sick from something you have not told me about." While this may sound adversarial, it really isn't. The people who make your food have an obligation to tell you what's in it at any given moment. Companies not willing to do this need another kind of attitude adjustment.

Attitude Adjustment No. 9
No one knows more about your problem than you do.

Understand that when it comes to your diet, no one is as clever, resourceful, or as smart. And no one has a better reason to be.

All too often, we sell ourselves short because we take the word of someone we presume to have authority. When the waiter tells us the chef uses flour to coat a cutlet or a plate of scallops, it's important to push past this immediate negative to the more palatable answer. Ask if that same dish can be prepared with rice flour or cornmeal or simply grilled or baked or roasted unadorned. With few exceptions, you will see the light bulb going on in the waiter's face. Remember, the chef is an expert on the preparation of food, not the preparation of *your* food.

And don't always assume your doctor knows more about living with your allergy or intolerance than you do. Most don't spend five minutes understanding the conditions they diagnose so expertly, especially if those conditions require no further medical intervention. If you need proof of this, ask your doctor for an opinion on kamut or spelt. The blank look should tell you everything you need to know.

I believe every one of us knows all we need to know in order to create our own happiness. It can be of enormous help if you try to believe this too. If the picture seems bleak, paint your own. Ask questions, make requests, switch dishes, start every sentence with "What if . . .," assume nothing, and trust that the other person can always say no. In my experience, very few ever do.

Attitude Adjustment No. 10
Never ask what is offered when you can tell what you need.

Call an airline and ask what foods are served on a gluten-free menu. Without too many exceptions, you will most likely hear about what won't be served. Call the same airline, tell them you are going to be flying to The Hague next month and that you need to have brown rice bread and wheat- or gluten-free cookies or cereal or muffins on board for your breakfast, and you may end up talking with the catering department and planning a meal. You may have to tell them where to get it too. But it sure beats the automatic no you get approaching them in the usual way. This applies to restaurants, hotels, spas, camps, hospitals, cruise ships, trains, and so on.

Remember it this way. In Washington, it's "ask, don't tell." In your life, it's "tell, don't ask."

Attitude Adjustment No. 11
People are basically good and decent.

If I sound like a hopeless idealist, I have learned that this is not necessarily a bad way to be. Yes, I know there are people who will mug you, steal your money, carjack your Ford Bronco, and, if you're not careful, deposit your life savings in their own Swiss accounts.

I'm not suggesting that you become foolish or naive, but I am suggesting that you give people the benefit of the doubt before you assume they are not interested in making your meals more pleasant.

If you're not sure, go to a public place such as a hospital or an office building and ask the receptionist if you can use the copy machine or phone simply by saying, "May I use your copy machine/ phone for a minute?" You may get lucky, but most likely you will be politely told to go to a stationery store or a phone booth.

Now go to another institution and ask the same question, this time starting with, "I hope you can help me. I really am in a tight spot and I wonder if you would be kind enough to allow me to make a copy of this/make a quick phone call." Chances are the person will offer to make the copies for you or hand you the phone.

The lesson is simple. The better your ability to ask a question in a way that encourages the other person to do the right thing, the better your chances of hearing the answer you want. The trick is asking it in a way that brings out the other person's natural instinct to help you. "You have no idea what a treat it would be for me to have your sauce on this pasta . . ."

Learning to do this is not so simple. Practice on your family.

"Darling, it would mean so much to me if you . . . took out the garbage, changed the cat's litter, passed that math test, lowered the stereo . . ."

CHAPTER FOUR

Dinner Is in the Mail

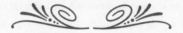

When it absolutely, positively has to be there overnight!
—FEDERAL EXPRESS COMMERCIAL

My next-door neighbor is hooked on shoes. She sits up at night and orders them in every imaginable design, fabric, price point, cultural persuasion, and elevation, from sporty to sensible, romantic and elegant to Frederick's of Hollywood sexy—sneakers, sling backs, boots, sandals, loafers, mules, ghillies, pumps, platforms, wedgies, spectators, clogs, combat boots, ballet slippers, oxfords, espadrilles, tennis shoes, high tops, huaraches, and heels so high, they cause nosebleeds in humans.

They arrive at the rate of about three pairs a week from fine stores all over the continental United States and beyond, often from such exotic locations as Paris and Milan. I know this because my neighbor is also a workaholic—how else could she afford this expensive pasttime?—and is never home to receive these enticing rectangular boxes.

Sonia, the UPS route person, doesn't even bother ringing my neighbor's bell. Knowing I work at home, she carries the new shoes to my door and we wonder aloud whether this latest pair will find a home or be returned. Nestled in their boxes, they sit on my hall bench, tissue paper in their toes, awaiting their new owner's verdict. I imagine I hear nervous tapping inside their shoe trees.

I think about my own parcels, which arrive at an equally steady clip, big cartons full of smaller packages of bread and cakes and cookies suspended in bubble wrap and cushioned in packing popcorn, releasing their own heady aromas of a dark and yeasty comfort far more primal and satisfying than the transient lure of fashion.

The woman in the brown UPS uniform is intrigued by her part in a "shoe thing," as she calls my neighbor's obsession, and wonders if I am ever tempted to consider a trade. We ponder the eternal question of how many pairs of shoes are enough for one person, and I think for a second, really just for appearances, because I know the answer without hesitation. There isn't a sole in all the closets of Ferragamo, Joan and David, Imelda Marcos, and the Fendi sisters combined that could compete with that perfect moment when my doorbell rings and Sonia sings out, "Bakery in a box for Mrs. Lowell!"

At my house, Christmas arrives pretty much once a month. It comes in a big carton filled with cookies, coffee cakes, muffins, linguini, fettuccine, angel hair pasta, lasagne, and gluten-free breads made with potato, rice, and tapioca flour. It takes the form of a velvety flourless cake named Decadence for good reason or a box of newly discovered macaroons I can't wait to try, and it appears in boxes of pancake, corn bread, muffin, cake, brownie, biscotti, and even bagel mixes that can be stirred, whirred, whisked, and baked into morsels that defy distinguishing them from "the real thing."

When I least expect it, Sonia pulls up in her brown truck and hands me a tin of fragrant corn sticks spiked with jalapeño peppers from a small restaurant in Los Angeles, where the chef took pity on me when I visited with a mutual friend and now bakes some extra for me every now and then. Sometimes they're still warm because she is thoughtful and ships them to me Overnight Express. When the doorbell rings again, I am in receipt of the breakfast I thought I could never have. I sign Sonia's clipboard with a trembling hand, the other clutching my brand-new bagel mix.

Happily, mail order is no longer the hit-or-miss proposition it once was. With space-age, airtight, refrigerated, heat-containing, and shelf-stable packages, UPS, Federal Express, DHL, and even Next Day Delivery from Uncle Sam, it is likely the blueberry muffins you had flown in from hundreds, maybe even thousands of miles away are still sticky and tender from the oven. In fact, with the help of a twenty-four-hour phone or fax order department most companies make available today, it is not outside the realm of possibility for those fudge brownies you couldn't stop thinking about last night to arrive in time for lunch or, at the very latest, for your afternoon nibble.

Sooner or later, though, you will receive moldy bread, soggy cookies, or something inedible. Most reputable mail-order companies will replace the products and reship with no additional cost and very little inconvenience to you. For this reason, it is wise to establish an account with your regular suppliers. I haven't found a company yet that refused to make good on something I didn't like or that arrived less than fresh.

Mail order is never inexpensive. If you insist on a "rush" order or if the product you are ordering is fragile and needs to be shipped overnight or second-day air to avoid arriving in a puddle, the freight charges can be hefty. For this reason, it always pays to order in quantity. When you do, though, remember to ask how long a product will keep, in the refrigerator, unopened on a shelf, or in the freezer without losing its appeal—whether that package is truly shelf stable or not. If it's an everyday item, such as bread or bread mix, and can be stored in the package for some time, it pays to buy in as much bulk as you have shelf space in order to keep the shipping costs down.

While there is no definitive IRS position on this fine point, it wouldn't hurt to ask your accountant or the IRS if the deductible cost of your doctor-prescribed food, provided that food is not available within a reasonable distance, includes shipping.

Although it would be impossible to list all the mail-order food companies that might carry a wheat- or gluten-free item, the following represent my favorite mail-order food companies. They've been unearthed through years of trial and error, discovery and disappointment—which, I warn you, will happen to you as well. Many of these companies are small and, for various reasons—taking on more than they can chew among the most notable—do not survive. There is only one thing worse than finding out a company you love is gone, and that's giving up the search for its replacement. The following people were all up and running at this printing. Although I wish I could be, I can't be responsible for changes of address, phone numbers, or ingredients, but for totally selfish reasons, I hope this book will do its part in keeping all of these good people in the black and strong.

Other companies come courtesy of Elaine Monarch and the Celiac Disease Foundation in Los Angeles, California, an information source whose number is listed in chapter 12 and should be transferred to your "A" list. Still others, new and untried, come from unexpected sources, the upfront "feature" pages of "food" magazines, newspaper articles, local celiac support group networking, American Celiac Society Dietary Support Coalition, Gluten Intolerance Group, and Celiac Sprue Association/USA newsletters, a wonderful gourmet guide to regional foods compiled by Allison and Margaret Engel called *Food Finds* (HarperCollins, 1991), and good old-fashioned word of mouth.

So many calories, so little time.

Allspice
734 South Ninth Street
Philadelphia, PA 19147
(215) 629-1904

I can walk over to Philadelphia's Italian market and have one of Mary Carrol's giant, freshly baked, maple syrup–sweetened, wheat- or gluten-free blueberry, corn, strawberry corn, chocolate espresso, pumpkin chocolate chip, or carrot raisin muffins any time I like. Even better, I can slap the screen door of this tiny corner bakery and remember what it was like to know the neighborhood baker and to stop and smell the flours, which in this case is pure soy. I am fortunate to have such treats so close to home. A working telephone and the will to eat healthfully are all you need for Mary to ship her low-fat goodies to you. You'll have to imagine the screen door. Minimum order ½ dozen, $9, single flavors or mixed. Check or money order only.

Authentic Foods
6333 W. Third Street, No. 742
Los Angeles, CA 90036
(213) 934-0424

Steven Rice makes a mean bean flour. It's made from a combination of garbanzo and fava beans, then ground into flour through a special process developed and perfected by this master chef himself, who believes there is a big difference between a substitute and a good-for-you alternative. Firm believer in the latter, this unusual chef dares anyone to match his unique flour for its healthful properties or its binding qualities, especially with chocolate, and proves it with a supermoist chocolate cake mix.

Bean flour, as well as the less exotic brown rice flour, can be purchased separately for independent experimentation, but I would advise taking advantage of years of trial and error with Steven's own falafel, bean burger, and pancake, muffin, and white bread mixes. An individual 1-pound package of mix will run approximately $2.80, and most products can be ordered by the case. Baking ingredients—vanilla powder, maple sugar, and xanthan gum—are also available through Authentic Foods' distributor, Thomas Mace & Associates, P.O. Box 898, Dana Point, CA 92629-0898, (800) 692-7323. Check, MasterCard, and Visa accepted.

B. P. Gourmet
295 Robbins Lane
Syosset, NY 11791
(516) 931-6620

This company makes wonderful wheat- and gluten-free, raisin-studded nuggets called Clusters in Chocolate or Vanilla and bite-size meringues called Dreams, which are concocted in flavors such as Cocoa, Chocolate Fudge, Milky Way, Lemon Meringue, and Chocolate Peanut Butter and are sometimes crisp, sometimes chewy, depending on the climate where they are stored. There are also crunchy miniatures called Rocky Road in Vanilla, Chocolate, Black Raspberry, Chocolate Apricot, and Chocolate Cheesecake. I love them, not only because they're good, but—grab your socks—all but Rocky Road are low calorie and fat-free! Minimum order is one case of twelve bags for $32, including shipping and two flavors if you like. Not to worry, you could eat a whole case of these while dialing. These and other cookies by B. P. Gourmet can be found in specialty markets around the country and not all are wheat- and gluten-free. Read all labels carefully before purchasing. Check or money order only.

Butte Creek Mill
402 N. Royal
P.O. Box 561
Eagle Point, OR 97524
(503) 826-3531
Fax (503) 830-8444

I discovered Butte Creek Mill's stone-ground cornbread mix at Dean & DeLuca in New York City, but you can order it direct from the mill. Other freshly milled gluten-free flours include yellow corn, soya, brown rice, and yellow and white cornmeal. Yellow corn grits and long- and short-grain whole-grain brown rice are other wheat-free alternatives. If you ever get to Oregon, check out Butte Creek Mill. Listed on the National Register of Historic Places, the mill is 123 years old at this printing. In the meantime, call or write for the product and price list. Visa and MasterCard accepted.

Dietary Specialties, Inc.
P.O. Box 227
Rochester, NY 14601
(800) 544-0099

I've been making Dietary Specialties layer cakes for years. I call them "Donna Reed" cakes because they're very fifties and they taste like life did before it got complicated. Donna always had a fresh one in the kitchen on every show, and for years I believed all grown women did all day was fiddle with icing, cut slices, and shoo greedy husbands, neighbors, and children away from their creations.

I fiddle with them too, but I add extra chocolate, shredded coconut, or jam between the layers. I even managed to turn one into a very festive birthday cake with the help of a nozzle, a pastry tube, and some whipped cream. I've drizzled chocolate syrup and stirred chocolate chips into the white cake mix for uneven but delicious results and used the mix for my wheat-free, gluten-free version of strawberry shortcake. (None of my guests suspected.) I must say Dietary Specialties brownie mix is much improved by the addition of extra chocolate and walnuts or pecans. I sometimes serve the brownies with scoops of ice cream, and if I'm feeling thin that day, I'll glaze them with fudge or butterscotch.

The people at Dietary Specialties are masters of the wheat- and gluten-free mix, and their products are a must to keep on hand for emergencies, especially if your schedule doesn't allow making these things from scratch and the child (real or imagined) in your family misses good old-fashioned mix cake with lots of gooey icing. Go easy, though, because gluten-free does not mean calorie- and fat-free.

Dietary Specialties also carries hard-to-find baking supplies such as gluten-free flavored extracts, xanthan and guar, rice crumb and exotic flours, condiments and spices, Maine blueberry and wild strawberry vinaigrette dressings, and a wheat- or gluten-free barbecue sauce and Oriental marinade I use at home and generously supply to friends for my backyard appearances at their grills.

Like their competition in Seattle, the Dietary Specialties product list boggles the mind. So what if the names of some of their products are a little strange? Anybody with a disease called celiac really shouldn't throw stones.

Among the offerings are Bi-Aglut Crackerbread; Vitamite non-dairy beverage mix; Aproten low-protein and gluten-free macaroni products, noodles, and pastas; Drei Pauly spaghetti and spirals; Papapasta lentil tagliatelle, lasagne, and angel hair; Papasnax plain salted, garlic, sesame, cumin, black pepper, and extra black pepper crackers; mixes for white or chocolate layer cake, and for brownies, blueberry or bran muffins, and brown bread.

There are flours, extracts, baking ingredients, and cookies—chocolate, vanilla, shortcake, wafers filled with vanilla or chocolate cream, custard cream, chocolate chip, or granola style.

Also available are Bette Hagman's wonderful books, *The Gluten-Free Gourmet* (Holt, 1990) and *More from the Gluten-Free Gourmet* (Holt, 1993).

Products are sold by the unit or by the case. Returns must be authorized (call 716 263-2787 first, *then* UPS). Check, money order, MasterCard, and Visa are accepted, and phone orders will be taken between 8:30 A.M. and 5 P.M. Eastern Standard Time. Your signature on record will really expedite things.

Ener-G Foods, Inc.
5960 1st Avenue South
P.O. Box 84487
Seattle, WA 98124
800-331-5222
Fax: (206) 767-4088

You may have already seen these products on your health food store's shelves. Ener-G Foods caters to wheat-free, gluten-free, low-protein, low-sodium, and lactose-restricted diets. There is very little you can't have for which this company hasn't already figured out how to make a reasonably good substitute. It will not only ship the foods you order, it also will provide a complete list and specific details of all its product's ingredients at your request.

I adore its Dutch cocoa cookies. They are dense, chocolatey, and utterly satisfying for eating whole, dunking, or rolling into a really good pie or cheese cake crust. I substitute the ginger cookies for the graham crackers in pie crusts. I cook the extra-wide noodles, leaving them a little more al dente than the package suggests, and layer them with mozzarella, ricotta, bits of chicken or vegetables, and fresh tomato sauce for a lasagne that rivals any I'd eaten in the days before diagnosis.

Ener-G Foods breads arrive in shelf-stable packages, so you can order in quantity. These people will not only make good on spoilage, they will do so with a smile you can feel through their 800 line.

Check, money order, Discover, MasterCard, Visa, and American Express are all acceptable methods of payment. Prices do not include shipping, and orders are sent UPS surface whenever possible. Toll-free numbers are in operation Monday through Friday, 8:30 A.M. to 5 P.M. Pacific Standard Time, and this company provides clear, written instructions for returns. It will also provide a list of recipes for your particular restriction—gluten-free, wheat-free, milk-free, soy-free, egg-free, no sugar added, corn-free, gelatin-free, among others—and will do so in French, if necessary, which I suspect is an outgrowth of bilingual Canada, where wheat and gluten intolerance is common. *Merci*, Ener-G.

New products are always being added to Ener-G's extensive inventory and existing ones are periodically reformulated, and I am rooting for them to get it right in the packaged bread department. With smaller companies developing truly wonderful breads and bread mixes, I personally think it's time for Ener-G to revamp their offerings which, for my money, come up short on taste and texture. For now, the following list should give you a general idea of the scope of this important resource.

Breads: white rice, tapioca, brown rice, brown rice potato, xanthan, poi, rice starch, egg, yeast-free white rice, yeast-free brown rice, and rice and fiber. Also available are white rice, tapioca or brown rice hamburger buns, white rice or tapioca hot dog buns, tapioca dinner rolls, rice bran muffins, blueberry muffins, rice pizza shells, broken Melba toast, croutons, stuffing bread crumbs, pie shells and tart shells.

Baked goodies: cinnamon rolls; fruitcake; cinnamon crackers; chocolate crisps; plain, banana, pumpkin, and apple-flavor doughnuts; almond butter, carob, chocolate, chocolate chip, Dutch cocoa, chocolate sandwich, sugar-free date, lemon sandwich, lemon shortbread, macaroon, orange, peanut butter, pumpkin, spice, walnut, and vanilla cream-filled wafer cookies.

Wheat- and gluten-free mixes and hard-to-find ingredients: corn bran, potato starch, potato flour, rice mix, low-sodium rice mix, brown rice baking mix, quick mix, brown or white rice flour, rice starch, rice polish, rice bran, tapioca flour, egg replacer, brown rice pilaf, methylcellulose, xanthan gum, baking powder, dry vinegar, baking soda or salt substitute, and wheat- but not gluten-free barley, oat, rice 'n' rye, oat bran, and millet.

And that's only the beginning. There are cereals, pastas, milk powders and milk substitutes, soup mixes, crackers, soup and salad seasonings, and allergy cookbooks.

It's best to open an account and get yourself a customer number.

The Famous Pacific Dessert Company
2414 SW Andover Street, C
Seattle, WA 98106-1100
(800) 666-1950
Fax (206) 935-2535

Chocolate cake as an art form. This company's Chocolate Decadence is really a flourless torte made with nothing but butter, sugar, cream, and the finest chocolate money can buy. It's unbelievably rich, expensive, and worth every bite. A 9-inch cake serves 12 to 16 people for $21; the 6-inch cake serves 6 to 8 for $15.50; and 4-ounce "mini-tortes" are $3.95 each. Puddle a 15-ounce jar of their locally grown Raspberry Puree around the bottom of the cake to cut the chocolate's richness. You may spend $12 for UPS second-day delivery, but you're definitely talking special occasion.

The torte is made with no preservatives or alcohol and comes in its own sealed, airtight plastic case. The company says it will keep without refrigeration for up to six months. I can't imagine anyone having the willpower to see if this is true. My favorite serving suggestion: a surprise "mini" gift wrapped and tucked into the lunch box of a very special birthday child or the briefcase of one who still is a child at heart. Phone orders and major credit cards are accepted.

If you ever get to Seattle, taste the Dacquoise, a frilly rosette-strewn confection made of meringue, ground hazelnuts, chocolate butter cream, powdered sugar, and a tiny bit of rum. It's too fragile to be shipped.

Food for Life Baking Company
2991 East Doherty Street
Corona, CA 91719
(909) 279-5090

Whenever I traveled West, I loaded up on this company's carrot and banana muffins, which made a real mess in my suitcase. Now it ships its wheat- and gluten-free products anywhere in the continental United States. Also available are gluten-free elbow pasta, and rice, rice almond, and brown rice breads. In the wheat-free-only department, look for millet, spelt, and white rye breads; plain, oatmeal, oat bran, and blueberry muffins; carob brownies; and blueberry cake. Check or money order only.

G! Foods
3536 Seventeenth Street
San Francisco, CA 94110
(415) 255-2139

This company's ad says, "I can't believe it's really" biscotti. Believe it. Randy Galterio and partner Lewis Gartenberg have created traditional Italian biscotti that are crisp, not too sweet, wheat- and gluten-free, and eminently dunkable. They arrive in such flavors as Almond, Chocolate-Chip Almond, Coconut Almond Chocolate-Chip, Hazelnut, and Chocolate-Chip Hazelnut. These authentic biscotti are sweetened with organic maple syrup and made with organically grown rice flour and eggs from "healthy" hens that have not been given any nasty antibiotics or hormones. No assembly required. Just put on a pot of espresso, open the box, and dunk. Better still, carry these to your favorite café and pull up a sidewalk. Also available are melting butter cookies in assorted flavors, seasonal and holiday assortments, fruity Date & Nut Breakfast Bars, and ingredients such as xanthan gum, gluten-free extracts and cookie crumbs for home baking.

Cookies are $12 for a 1-pound bag, $6.26 for a ½-pound bag in single flavors or mixed assortments, or come individually wrapped, 1 pound for $14 or $1.25 each. Single portions are ideal for traveling, the office, picnic baskets, glove compartments, and fit nicely into the average purse. Phone and credit card orders are accepted, and a ½-pound trial sampler pack is $10 including shipping.

The Gluten-Free Pantry
P.O. Box 881
Glastonbury, CT 06033
(203) 633-3826

Beth Hillson, celiac, mother of a celiac, food and travel writer, and the owner of, chef for, and creative force behind this gluten-free, gourmet food company, has divined one of the best mail-order mixes I have ever tasted. Her bagels were the toast of *Good Morning, America*. Her truffle brownies are sinfully rich, and her white bread mix rivals any for the authentic taste and texture of the real thing. You will find a few of her incredible recipes in chapters 10 and 11.

She sells mixes for caraway "rye" bread, brioche, challah, chocolate chip cookies and squares, orange walnut biscotti, cranberry orange bread, buttermilk brown rice pancakes, sugar cookies, and a new French bread/pizza. There is even a gluten home test kit that will pick up minute particles of wheat and other grains in home foods; at $49.50, it beats the cost of hiring a taster. Prices range from $3.95 to $5.95 per 1-pound bag with a 10 percent discount on cases. No special baking skills are required for these products, and a bread machine is nice but not necessary. All major credit cards are accepted. Put this number on speed dial.

Goodie's on Melrose
7217 Melrose Avenue
Los Angeles, CA 90046
(213) 934-3001

Jo Ann Ross Harvey, the owner of this unusual, gluten-free bakery on L.A.'s trendy Melrose Avenue, is allergic to yeast as well as to wheat and gluten and several other foods. She has managed to turn that liability into a major asset, creating desserts not to die for, but to live for in the healthiest possible sense. Her cookies are fabulous—so good, in fact, that my Los Angeles friends have a hard time not polishing off the supply they lay in for my trips west before I even arrive. The chocolate chip cookies and peanut butter delights are soft and chewy, just the way you remember them, and the orange, strawberry, blueberry, and cinnamon walnut morsels are equally satisfying.

Also available are frosted cupcakes, coffee cakes, cinnamon streusel coffee cake, and lemon ricotta cheese rollovers from this ingenious baker who decided she too needed to go "against the grain" to get what she wanted. Eating at this unusual bakery is an experience, but short of a personal appearance, a valid credit card and a telephone will get you your own supply. Prices range from $2.50 to $3.25 for a ¼ pound. Gift baskets, boxes, and tins are available, and Visa, MasterCard, American Express, and Diner's Club International are all accepted.

The King's Cupboard
P.O. Box 27
Red Lodge, MO 59068
(800) 962-6555
Fax (406) 446-3070

The people here make the best chocolate sauces ever to be drizzled over a scoop of ice cream, blanketed a strawberry into, or just plain licked off the spoon. They use no artificial colorings, preservatives, stabilizers, or flavorings, only fresh cream, local butter, dark unsweetened chocolate, cocoa, and sugar. But they do use vanilla, which makes them off-limits to those of you who are very sensitive.

There is Bittersweet Chocolate, Espresso Chocolate, and Orange Chocolate in 10-ounce jars at $8.95 or 4.5-ounce jars at $4.95, which does not include shipping. Prepaid Visa and MasterCard orders only.

Kingsmill Foods Company Ltd.
1339 Kennedy Road
Scarborough, Ontario MIP 2L6

No kidding, this company makes "UNIMIX," a low-protein, all-in-one, gluten-free mix that will make a loaf, buns, cookies, pizza, pasta, doughnuts, and Melba toast. It's the "play dough" of mixes and the brainchild of the faculty of Food Sciences at the University of Toronto. For $2 and a money order, you can try it. Kingsmill also sells canned bread, cookies, baking ingredients, and pastas. No credit cards. No phone orders.

Lundberg Family Farms
P.O. Box 369
Richvale, CA 95974
(916) 882-4551

These are the people with whom to enjoy a nice, hot breakfast. They'll ship rice cereal, and they also make rice cakes, brown rice, rice blends, pudding mixes, and something they call Riz-cous for the authentic Moroccan recipes you've been afraid to try until now. No credit cards. Check or money order only.

Nature's Hilights
P.O. Box 3608
Chico, CA 95927
(800) 828-8828

If you're wondering what happened to the people who make the frozen wheat- and gluten-free brown rice pizzas, pizza shells, and tostadas formerly called Snack Cracks, wonder no more. They've changed their name. You still have to look for their pizzas in the health food store, but they'll ship their breadsticks anywhere in the continental U.S. as long as you have a major credit card.

Pamela's Products
156 Utah Avenue
South San Francisco, CA 94080
(415) 952-4546

You may have seen these cookies on the shelves of your health food store. If not, you can send for these buttery morsels in peanut butter, ginger, butter shortbread, cocoa shortbread, chunky chocolate chip, chocolate double chip, carob hazelnut, or pecan shortbread, each $3 for an 8-ounce package.

Other wheat- and gluten-free items available are coconut macaroons; soya cupcakes; Pamela's ultra chocolate brownie mix with chocolate chips; Mrs. Leeper's vegetable corn pastas; baking mixes with recipes for pizza crust, pie, pancakes, and waffles; and a good selection of hard-to-find gluten-free puddings and wheat-free cookies in two flavors, oatmeal raisin walnut and oatmeal date coconut. A catalog is available. Checks or money orders only. Shipping outside California costs $1 extra; $7 extra for Hawaii and Alaska.

The Really Great Food Company
P.O. Box 319
Malverne, NY 11565
(516) 593-5587

The mailer for this company says it uses special varieties of rice for its flours, which are then specially processed to open the starch grains and allow the mixes to bake up lighter than the typical, heavy-textured gluten-free products. Personally, I think it's because the partners also happen to be celiacs and developed the mixes for themselves first. Whatever the reason, their dark, moist gingerbread muffin mix is "really great," to quote a company slogan—so good, in fact, you might not be able to tell the difference.

This company also makes "really great" wheat- and gluten-free cornbread, pancake, muffin, cookie, pizza crust mixes, and even a basic one that can be used as a substitute for regular wheat- and gluten-free flour in recipes. There are also brown rice elbows, fusilli, spirals, and spaghetti that the partners say tastes just like wheat in 9-

ounce, two-portion packages. I would say this is a "really great" resource for anyone with recent memories of the real thing.

Prices do not include shipping via UPS and range from $1.35 for a 13-ounce package of cornbread mix to $6.50 for a 3-pound bag of white flour pancake mix. Checks or money orders only. Allow two to four weeks for delivery.

Red Mill Farms
290 South 5th Street
Brooklyn, NY 11211
(718) 384-2150
Fax (718) 384-2988

This is the home of Jennie's Macaroons, those gluten-free, lactose-free, individually wrapped coconut goodies found near the checkout counter in many markets and health food stores. Red Mill also makes gluten- and lactose-free Dutch chocolate and banana nut "cake-in-a-can" not sold in stores. They started out being made for Passover and for people who could remember what regular cake tasted like and who could go back to the real thing after the holidays. Single or case orders are accepted. Prices range from $4 to $54. Check or money order only. No shipping charge for one-case orders.

Shiloh Farms
438 White Oak Road
New Holland, PA 17557
(800) 829-5100

The folks here, who distribute their products under the name Garden Spot, make wonderful cookie, muffin, waffle, and loaf mixes that substitute cup for cup for the wheat flour in most recipes. They will also ship pizza crust mix or pound cake mix, or bake it for you in the form of cinnamon raisin rice bread, white rice bread, and rolls. Beans, seeds, dried fruits, and allowable grains and flours are among the many offerings in their extensive catalog, which breaks down products for dairy-free, salt-free, wheat-sensitive, wheat-free, yeast-free, vegetarian, and gluten-free diets. Phone orders and Visa or MasterCard are accepted.

Starbucks Coffee Company
2203 Airport Way South
Post Office Box 34510
Seattle, WA 98124
(800) 782-7282

   The people who perk the trendiest and best coffee on the planet
also offer a mean Chocolate Espresso Mousse Cake. Described in the
Starbucks catalog as being totally flourless, this meltingly rich concoction of bittersweet chocolate, butter, sugar, eggs, cocoa, and espresso
is said to be "a slice of heaven." They're not kidding. I say, why buy
a slice when you can have the whole heavenly deal (8-inch, 1 pound,
4 ounces), for $29.95 plus shipping? While you're at it, order some
coffee to wash it down and start a petition to get this cake on the
menu in the Starbucks cafés that seem to be popping up everywhere
these days. MasterCard, Visa, American Express, check or money order accepted.

Walnut Acres
Penns Creek, PA 17862
(800) 433-3998

   The ad says "healthful, delicious organic foods delivered to your
door," and the catalog alone is worth a phone call. Vitamins, books,
bakeware, utensils, fruit spreads, chemical-free vegetables, juices,
fruits, all-natural peanut and almond butters, nuts, fruit and nut mixes
as well as wheat-free grains, grits, mixes, whole-grain rices, rice blends
of every exotic hue, soy and goat milk powders, even ghee, the clarified butter used in Indian cooking. Visa, MasterCard and Discover
cards. Check and money order accepted.

Wel-Plan
Anglo-Dietetics, Ltd.

   Sounds like an HMO, doesn't it? The brochure says the products
are "for patients on gluten-free, low-protein or allergen-free diets." So
what if they haven't figured out that we're not sick, we're customers? I
can live with that.

   No prescription is necessary to order brown or white bread mix;
canned brown bread; soya bran; baking mix; cream-filled vanilla or

chocolate wafers; custard cream, raisin, chocolate, or savory cookies; macaroni or spaghetti.

These products have an extended shelf life and can be ordered through Dietary Specialties (see page 76).

Williams-Sonoma—A Catalog for Cooks
Mail Order Department
P.O. Box 7456
San Francisco, CA 94120
(800) 541-2233
Fax: (415) 421-5153

The one and only "Williecake Collection." According to the catalog, these flourless confections were created by Chef Willing Howard in honor of his young son, but all you need to know is this: Belgian bittersweet chocolate, Dutch cocoa powder, butter, sugar, rum, and fresh eggs, no nasty artificial colorants, emulsifiers, extenders, preservatives or added salt and that's just original Chocolate. There's Espresso (full of crunchy coffee beans), Raspberry, and Grand Marnier, and not a bit of wheat or gluten in sight. $36 plus shipping via air in a cold pack will get you a 7-inch chocolate torte that serves 10 to 12. $38 for the other flavors. Check, money order, and major credit cards accepted. Gift certificates are available.

You're going to use a lot of rice and corn. Why not become a connoisseur? Skip the sticky supermarket varieties and do some homework by mail. Order grains freely, but *never* assume an advertised mix is wheat- or gluten-free. Ask first, then go wild, as in rice from these companies.

Gibbs Wild Rice
10400 Billings Road
Live Oak, CA 95953
(800) 824-4932
No credit cards accepted.

Guillory's Popcorn Rice
Louisiana Rice Company
Route 3, Box 55
Welsh, LA 70591
(318) 734-2251 or (318) 734-4440
Credit cards are accepted with a minimum purchase of $10.

McFadden Farm Wild Rice and Dried Herbs
Potter Valley, CA 95469
(800) 544-8230

Minnesota Specialty Crops
69 Airport Boulevard
McGregor, MN 55760
(800) 328-6731

Northern Lakes Wild Rice Company
P.O. Box 592
Teton Village, WY 83025
(307) 733-7192
No credit cards accepted.

St. Maries Wild Rice
P.O. Box 293
St. Maries, ID 83861
(208) 245-5835

For yellow or blue cornmeal, corn flour, grits, and polenta, in addition to many of the companies already listed, contact:

Edward's Mill
The School of the Ozarks
Point Lookout, MO 65726
(417) 334-6411
No credit cards accepted.

Gray's Grist Mill
P.O. Box 422
Adamsville, RI 02801
(508) 636-6075
Credit cards are accepted with a $25 minimum.

Josie's Best New Mexican Foods, Inc.
P.O. Box 5525
Santa Fe, NM 87502
(505) 983-6520
Blue corn flour, blue cornmeal; no credit cards accepted.

Kenyon Corn Meal Company
Usquepaugh, RI 02892
(401) 783-4054

Lakeside Mills
Route 1, Box 38
Seven Springs, NC 28578
(919) 569-0111
No credit cards accepted.

Mallard Pond Farms
746 Mallard Pond Drive
Boulder, CO 80303
(303) 494-3551
Unique gluten-free popcorn flour.

Tuthilltown Grist Mill
1020 Albany Post Road
Gardiner, NY 12525
(914) 255-5695
No credit cards or telephone orders accepted.

And for those wheat-free "onlys" who can tolerate it:

Christine & Rob's Oatmeal
41103 Stayton-Schio Road
Stayton, OR 97383
(503) 769-2993

For those of you who do something other than go to the beach or attend luaus on vacation in Hawaii:

Chong's Poi Shop
P.O. Box 1753
Kaunakakai, Molokai, HI 96748
(808) 553-5824

Mail-order Homework

There are many other wonderful wheat- and gluten-free foods to be found on the pages of magazines, especially city magazines that promote local businesses, in newspaper articles, in special advertising sections mailers, in free papers in markets and health food stores, and even along the side of the road at farm stands, independent bakeries, candy shops, mills, even malls. The trick is to look, make phone calls, ask questions, tell people why you need to know, and understand that many businesses have no idea their products are important to people like you until you tell them. Some will ship and others that are too small may make an exception in your case. Whenever you travel, make finding new resources a challenge. Don't just walk into a store and buy what you came in for. Look around, chat, ask questions, discover the joy of serendipity, and add it to your growing knowledge that living "against the grain" means living in the constant expectation of knowing what you need is just around the next corner or right in front of you. All you have to do is be open to it and look.

The following handful of companies should get you started, but only that. I haven't even begun to list all the wheat- and gluten-free goodies yet to be found just beyond the porch of a country store or in the willingness of a chef or a wizard with flour. The perfect praline, the most sinful truffle, the hottest mustard, and the person who bakes a pie that will send you straight to heaven are still out there just around the bend. You need to discover these yourself because in doing so, you will find the gift of your own resourcefulness as well, which will serve you long after the UPS truck and the last cookie are gone. Let me know how you do.

Goldwater's Foods of Arizona
P.O. Box 9846
Scottsdale, AZ 85253
(800) 488-4932
The senator's own salsas and chili seasonings.

Hallam's Peanut Butter
P.O. Box 700
Nixa, MO 65714
(417) 725-2601
Homemade, pure, no preservatives.

St. Julien Macaroons
White Oak Farms Inc.
13 Lake Street
Sherborn, MA 01770
(508) 653-5953
Information on celiac sprue on request. No credit cards accepted.

Summer Garden Vinaigrettes
W. J. Clark & Co.
5400 W. Roosevelt Road
Chicago, IL 60650
(800) 229-0090
Wheat- and gluten-free salad dressings and marinades.

CHAPTER FIVE

Restaurant Assertiveness Training

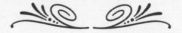

You can't always get what you want,
but if you try some time,
you just might find
you get what you need.

—THE ROLLING STONES

If you're like most people on severely restricted diets, when someone mentions eating out, you have serious reservations.

You imagine a cleaver-wielding chef pronouncing "No substitutions!" You cower before menus full of buffalo wings, fried mozzarella, meat loaf, and biscotti. Whole columns of pizza spin before you, and you speed-read through breakfasts, lunches, and dinners, desserts, appetizers, à la carte items, side dishes, late-night snacks, and take-out looking for the one thing you can order and actually enjoy.

You briefly consider a burger, but the sight of it, stripped of its processed cheese, white vinegar–laced mustard, and equally suspicious ketchup, sitting alone on your plate, denied the plump comfort of its bun, is too horrible, and you reconsider. You decide on a salad sprinkled with a little oil, lemon, and wine vinegar. Boring, but safe.

If you are not prepared, dining out can be a supremely unsatisfying experience. Certain meals are exquisite torture for the wheat and gluten intolerant, such as brunch with its muffins and croissants, sweet rolls and Danish pastries. If that were not bad enough, the problem often is compounded by having to explain your diet twice—first to the waiter, who must be sufficiently convinced that you are no mere faddist who believes eliminating wheat and other grains from your diet will whittle your waistline, put you in touch with your past lives, or some other dietary foolishness before he or she will relay it to the chef, who, in turn, must understand completely. Something can go wrong in the translation. Even the crash and clatter of restaurant and kitchen acoustics can be trouble.

"The woman at table twenty is allergic to wheat."

"What?"

"Wheat!"

"Heat?"

"No, wheat!"

"No beets for table twenty!"

Are you ready to venture forth into the world of eating out? Will you be able make reservations without any of your own, hold your ground with a surly or overworked waiter, stand up for your rights as a customer, order fearlessly, have the chef eating out of your hand, and live to tell the tale? Take this simple multiple-choice quiz and find out.

THE RESTAURANT READINESS QUIZ
A Menu of Multiple Choices

1. You phone a hot new restaurant and a bored-sounding hostess says they won't be able to fit you in for at least six weeks. You . . .
  a. reserve a table anyway, knowing it will be even harder to get in once the place is reviewed.
  b. ask if they could possibly fit you in sooner.
  c. explain that you won't be hungry by then and make a reservation someplace friendlier.

2. You order a bowl of onion soup and discover a hunk of bread lurking under the melted cheese topping. You . . .
  a. ask the waiter to remove the bread and return the bowl to you.

   b. accept it as is and fish out the soggy bread yourself.
   c. find out what kind of cheese is used and ask that a fresh bowl
       be made using that cheese only.

   3. You ask for a side dish of rice instead of the spaghetti that
comes with the meal and the waiter says, "No substitutions." You . . .
   a. explain your problem and ask if the management is willing to
       make an exception in your case.
   b. order something you don't like and resolve not to patronize
       this establishment again.
   c. ask if that rule also applies to the business they're losing in you.

   4. You are considering a dish that derives its sauce from something called a "roux." You . . .
   a. don't want to expose your lack of culinary sophistication and
       order the dish anyway, assuming the sauce involves red wine.
   b. make a joke about not being accustomed to cheek color in your
       food and ask the waiter what this is.
   c. decide not to take any chances and order something less com-
       plicated.

   5. Your friends decide on the local Italian restaurant for the Friday
night get-together. You . . .
   a. are outnumbered and agree, figuring you'll have a good lunch
       and find something you can have.
   b. tell them you'd love to come, but you really have to sort out
       that pesky sock drawer.
   c. explain that if they really would like your company, they'll have
       to choose somewhere less difficult for you.
(For answers, see page 114.)

   If you're like most people, you need to do a little homework. With
some advance planning and a thorough understanding of how to make
reservations, read a menu, communicate with a waiter, stand firm,
speak up, be understood, make special requests, and, most important,
carry your own supplies, eating out can be the pleasure it once was,
the treat it should always be.
   From your first contact with the reservations person to the mo-

ment you ask for the check, there are some very specific ways to enhance your chances of having a truly satisfying experience in a restaurant. Most stem from these general rules that apply to any situation.

Jax's Rules of Order

1. Never discuss your requirements with the waiter unless you have his or her complete and undivided attention.

2. Never pretend you understand a menu term or method of preparation if you don't. Ask.

3. Never accept the waiter's best guess, however sincere. Insist on verification that what you are putting into your mouth is wheat- or gluten-free.

4. Always be willing to convey your request personally to whoever is preparing your food.

5. Never pay for what you can't eat. Even if it's no one's fault, send it back and tell the waiter why.

6. Be prepared to leave any establishment in which you are denied the attention and consideration you request and deserve.

Reservations

Phoning ahead has never been more important. Obviously, if you are planning a visit to a popular restaurant, you must make reservations. But even if you are dining at a casual, neighborhood place, it's smart and polite to call ahead anyway and use this first communication to establish your special requirements.

After you are asked the number of people in your party, the time and date of arrival, the smoking status of your table, et cetera, et cetera, take the opportunity to tell the manager that you have a serious problem with wheat or other specific grains. Here you must remember how much you knew about gluten before you were diagnosed and be careful never to use this word unless you want to sink deeper and deeper into the other person's ignorance. I usually say I am not allowed any grains except rice and corn, even the tiniest trace, in any form, and leave it at that. At this point, explain that you need to know a little about the menu. Ask what entrées and desserts you can anticipate having, given this restriction, and whether the chef is willing to make some changes and adaptations for you.

If the person taking your reservation is rude, dismissive, doesn't know the answers, or just doesn't get it, this is the time to ask to speak with the chef, but only if you are calling at a time of day when this is possible. Don't expect the busy chef to go over the entire menu with you, but do say something like "I'd really love to be able to come to your restaurant, but I can't eat wheat, or any grains except rice and corn, and I'm wondering if you would be kind enough to adjust a little for me when I am there?"

Never be defensive. The idea is to appeal to the artist as well as to the businessperson. Do say how hard it is for you to find foods you can eat and that you would love to be able to really enjoy his or her cooking and that you are looking for a restaurant and a chef with whom you can enjoy a frequent and regular relationship. At this point, the chef will probably rise to the challenge and say, "Don't worry, I'll make anything you like. Just let me know when you come in."

If this is an Italian restaurant and you are planning your dinner on a weeknight, this is the time to ask "If I bring you a box of my pasta, will you cook it for me and put one of your gorgeous sauces on it?" If asked this way, the chef will probably cook pasta for you on any night, but I suggest you not try this when the kitchen is busy. At peak hours, there is a much greater chance of having your pasta mixed up with the regular fare. Anyway, it's just plain bad manners to ask a well-timed, flawlessly choreographed professional kitchen to add an unplanned pot on a Friday or Saturday night.

In the fifteen years I have been making these requests, it is a rare chef who refuses to make something special for me. I think this is because people who cook for others are nurturing types who enjoy the challenge of solving a special problem and the reward of knowing a customer is truly happy, especially one who isn't often or easily rendered so. If you can get to the chef, you will probably find a kindred spirit and a willing spatula.

If it is not too far out of your way and the chef cannot, for good reason, come to the phone when you call, I suggest you visit the restaurant, preferably early in the day, to examine the menu and ask these questions in person before making a reservation. All too often a chef pops out of the kitchen just at the right moment and, before you know it, you're both planning your dinner. Serendipity? The chef may think so.

This may seem like an awful lot of trouble for one meal. And it is. But the idea isn't just eating, it's eating well, and besides, you're worth it. Of course, once you have made this personal contact with a person who is willing to cook for you, you will probably never have to explain your problem again, at least not in that restaurant.

If the establishment is not friendly to your request, either to speak personally with the chef or for special attention when you arrive, cancel the meal.

If you do cancel, make sure the restaurant knows why. Drop the owner a note registering your disappointment at not being able to enjoy the establishment because you were not made to feel welcome. By all means, mention the ten friends who would have been dining with you that night had you and your needs not been dismissed so summarily.

Chances are, the owner or chef has no idea of the reception customers are getting and will be grateful for the opportunity to make it up to you. Most people don't realize that in order to withstand the grueling hours and backbreaking work required in the restaurant business, one must truly love it. I have to believe, and my own experience supports this, that if given the chance, a professional chef and smart businessperson will always choose to do the right thing. Even if love doesn't drive that decision, competition certainly does.

Incidentally, if you're not the one in your circle to make reservations, now is the time to volunteer. You have more at stake than everyone else. Whoever makes the call calls the shots. It's that simple.

If you are one of those people who like to go along with the crowd, this is also the time to work on becoming more assertive. It really is better to say "If you don't mind, I'd really rather not go to Restaurant X because there isn't much there I can enjoy" rather than going along with a plan that excludes you. You may not intend to, but I promise you, you will sulk and make everybody at the table miserable. And worse, you will blame the people who suggested the restaurant instead of the one who agreed to it—you.

You wouldn't allow the maître d' to decide whether you will sit with smokers, so why leave your meal to chance and the whims of well-meaning friends? Never, under any circumstances, take pot luck. Don't have reservations, make them.

The Waiter

Most waiters are wonderful, eager, hardworking, and professional people who sincerely want you to enjoy yourself and leave a large tip. However, you cannot assume that just because someone is carrying a corkscrew and a towel, he or she has any understanding of your particular problem or even any reason to care.

As soon as you arrive, just after the menus are handed out and the initial seating chatter dies down, draw the waiter aside. Explain that you are going to need help ordering and that it may be necessary to ask the chef some important questions. Explain your problem as simply as you can in much the same way you explained it to the hostess and stress the importance of being sure of the answer. If you have already spoken to the chef during the reservation phase, now is the time to ask the waiter to announce your arrival to the kitchen. If you have brought some of your own food to fill in—rice bread, pasta, an individual pizza crust, rice crackers or toast—this is a good time to alert the waiter.

Whenever possible, involve the waiter in your problem and appeal to the person, not to the job description. Never snap your fingers. That's rude under any circumstances. Never shout your request across the table. Never explain your problem to the bus person. And never call the waiter "sir" or "miss." They're called waiters or wait persons. Use that term or their names if they've introduced themselves (which I think is silly and overly familiar, but that's just me).

Say things such as "I really need your help here. . . . I'm sure you wouldn't want me to become ill. . . . You know so much more about this menu than I. . . . Please check. If you are wrong, it would be very bad for me." Involve the waiter in the solution to the problem: "What if the chef used rice flour to dust the soft shell crabs or simply sautéed them without any flour at all?" "What if the chef made a pizza with my pizza shell?" "What if we put your sauce on this pasta?" "What if" is the operative phrase here.

Very few people realize, unless they've done it themselves, how hard on the feet waiting tables really is, so the important thing in getting the waiter in your corner, or at your table, to be more precise, is to warn him or her that some extra trips to the kitchen on your behalf might be necessary. It's hard to resent extra work you can plan for and a customer who treats you with understanding and respect. Empathy. There's nothing like it for getting what you want.

You may be the most solicitous customer ever born, but you occasionally will run into trouble. It is inevitable, so you may as well be prepared.

The Difficult Waiter

Even though we should have known better, some months ago my friend Jim and I lunched at a pricey and altogether pretentious restaurant that shall, for these purposes, remain nameless. We were attended by the kind of waiter who never smiles and implies with every syllable that he would dearly love to be doing anything else but waiting on you. To get even for the fact that you are sitting at the table and not he, he does all he can to insure that your meal becomes a vehicle for social torture and public humiliation. You know the type.

My friend is not an unsophisticated eater and he does know his way around a good menu, but he is fond of ketchup on certain foods, an idiosyncracy no doubt left over from too many prep schools and summers at camps where meals were served from steam tables and everything tasted like damp wool.

When Jim requested a dollop of the stuff for his Fiddlehead Fern and Feta or some other equally dumb name for an omelette, our waiter rose to his full height and said in the most condescending tone possible, "I'm sorry, sir, but our chef does not believe in ketchup."

People believe in God, or in euthanasia, or in the death penalty, or even in a free market economy, but they don't believe in condiments. I waited for my pal, who has been known to explode an ego or two with a well-chosen word, and relished what was to come. To my surprise,

Jim's response was a meek "Oh, I see." The conversation turned to other matters and the moment was forgotten, or so I thought.

After a long, chatty meal over which we dallied far more than usual and out of spite, I suspect, we ordered espresso. The waiter returned with our coffees and a bowl of sugar options all in little packets. Just as he was about to turn on his heel, Jim crooked a finger and summoned the man back. Noticeably stung from this treatment, but eager to add to his earlier victory, the waiter tapped his pepper mill and wore a look of pure scorn.

"Tell me," Jim said, looking smartly down his nose at the pink packets of sugar substitutes, "what is your chef's position on aspartame?"

Okay. So you don't think like Noel Coward and sound like Maggie Smith. No matter what you do, the difficult waiter will always be difficult. But you, dear one, may take comfort in the fact that you will always be the customer, and, as such, you will always have the last word, which may be no more than "thanks!" written sarcastically above a five-cent tip, but no less effective. Rudeness takes most people by surprise, so it helps to know the kinds of things difficult waiters probably will say and plan your responses ahead of time.

When someone who expects you to pay for a meal treats you badly, the rule is—take no prisoners. My pet peeve is the waiter who interrupts me in midsentence, just to announce, "I'm Richard and I'll be your waiter this evening." When this happens and I am in the mood, I cut right to the bottom line and say, "I'm so-and-so and I'll be responsible for your tip this evening, so I'd appreciate your waiting until I am finished talking to make your announcements." I realize not everyone is comfortable doing this, but it does serve to put things in perspective very quickly and lets you know what you're up against right from the start of the meal.

Use these only when reason and all else fails:

1. You have very carefully explained your problem and the importance of your need to know exactly what is in each dish you are considering. You know all of this has fallen on deaf ears when the

waiter laughs and says with an unmistakeable tisk in the voice, "Is this some kind of new diet?"

You say: "Yes, it is. It's the if-I-get-so-much-as-a-speck-of-grain-I'll-die-and-all-my-living-relatives-will-sue-you-diet."

2. You ask if there is any flour or grain in something you're thinking of ordering or, worse, it has already arrived and your dinner is inedible. You ask that it be taken back. Instead of a prompt response, you get a roll of the eyes, a look of undisguised annoyance, and the answer "It's only a little."

You say: "In that case, I'll only sue you a little."

3. You've been through all the desserts on the menu and every one of them is made with flour. Like the relative who tries to get off the hook by putting you on it, the difficult waiter often will try to solve the restaurant's problem by suggesting the now-familiar "Why don't you just eat the middle?"

You say: "Why don't I just pay for the middle too?"

The good news is this won't happen to you very often. But when it does, your response should be swift and to the point. Naturally, there will be witnesses, and it doesn't hurt to let people know you are not someone who suffers fools or rudeness well.

The Menu

Have you ever played a game called Dictionary, where one person picks a word from the dictionary and writes down its real meaning, while others invent meanings for the word? Papers are collected, mixed up, read, and a vote taken. Whoever guesses the real meaning wins the most points for that round.

It sounds as if it would be difficult to find a word at least one person did not know the meaning of, but there are thousands of words with which even the most educated of us aren't familiar. We just pretend we are or let them slip by until we have enough context to shape a meaning. Unfortunately, we do the same thing when we read menus.

By the time we understand the context, we've literally swallowed our pride. This is a particularly dangerous form of dietary Russian roulette. After taking the following crash course, your grasp of culinary terms most commonly found on a menu will amaze your friends and stun your enemies, while keeping you happily wheat- and gluten-free.

CULINARY TERMS

According to *Larousse Gastronomique,* a roux is a mixture of flour and a fatty substance, most commonly butter, which is cooked and used as a thickening element for sauces. A roux can be white, blond, or brown, depending on how it is prepared. No matter what color, it is to be avoided like the plague. The word *roux* is rarely seen on the menu itself, but waiters often use the term to describe a sauce. Listen carefully for it.

Many French sauces are based on this technique. Because of this, most are not wheat- and gluten-free unless the chef specifically tells you the roux has been omitted or prepared with rice flour. Many modern chefs have omitted this classic and artery-clogging step in the name of "nouvelle cuisine" and now rely on vegetable reductions for their sauces. Nevertheless, you can never go wrong asking for specific ingredients whenever you see the following sauces listed on the menu:

Africaine, Albert, Alboni, Allemande, Americaine, Anglais, Bechamel, Béarnaise, Bigarade, Bordelaise, Bourguignonne, Butter, Cardinal, Chateaubriand, Chaud-froid or Brown Sauce, Chausseur or Hunter, Diable, Lyonnaise, Madeira, Maître d'hotel, Moutarde, Mornay, Nantua, Provençal, Ravigote, Robert, Supreme, Soubise, Veron, Velouté, and plain old American White.

Classic Demi-Glace sauces are usually not made with flour and form the basis for many other sauces, including tomato coulis and Espagnole sauce, which can be made with fish or meat stock. Since many chefs pride themselves on the liberties they take with the classics, however, it is always better to be safe than wrong.

Watch out for mayonnaise-based Remoulade sauce, which also contains mustard, and Vinaigrette, which is based on vinegar and can be made with mustard as well.

In the words of that awful French woman, "Let them eat . . . baba, baguette, beignet, brioche, buche de noel, charlotte, choux, crepe, croissant, croquette, croustade, eclair, flan, fritters, galantine, galette, gateau, genoise, gougere, genoise, gnocchi, kugelhopf, kulich, macaroon, mazarin, napolitain, Napoleon, noiseine, nommette, noques, nougatine, pain, pain Anglais, panetone, pannequet, pâté, pavé, petits four, piroghi, praline, profiterole, quenelle, quiche, rotie, roule, savarin, St. Honoré, strudel, tarte, terrine, tourte, vacherin, and vol-au-vent, and oh, yes . . . cake." You can't.

But you *can* memorize this abbreviated glossary of foods the wheat and gluten intolerant must avoid:

Albondigas. Mexican fried meat cakes that usually contain flour.

Americaine. A tomato sauce once based on lobster coral, but now commonly thickened with the more plentiful wheat flour.

Arlesienne. A dish or garnish composed of fried eggplants and fried onion rings dredged in flour.

Au gratin. Translation: Floury cheese sauce and bread crumbs.

Beef Wellington. This dish is always served "en croute" or in a pastry crust that has been slathered with pâté. Forget it.

Beignet. A dessert fritter popular in Louisiana and restaurants specializing in Cajun cuisine.

Blanquette. A veal or chicken ragout or stew based on a white roux.

Bisque. A thick soup or puree commonly thickened with flour.

Bouchée. Any bite-size puff pastry that is filled with sweet or savory ingredients as a dessert or hors d'oeuvre.

Bourguignonne. A stew containing Burgundy wine and roux.

Couscous. A North African specialty usually made of crushed durum wheat or millet flour, chick peas, or rice and steamed with spices and lamb, mutton, or chicken.

Crepinette. A small, fat sausage encased in bread crumbs.

Croque monsieur. A grilled sandwich, usually ham and gruyère cheese.

Crouton. A small, buttered cube of dried bread usually served in salads and soups, often invisible until it ends up in your mouth.

Escabeche. A Spanish dish consisting of floured and fried smelts, mackerels, whitings, and red mullets.

Foccaccia. You don't care how it's made. It's bread.

Friccasee. A method of preparation or stew consisting of flour-thickened white sauce and poultry.

Frito misto. A traditional Italian dish of foods fried in flour and egg batter.

Gnocchi. Italian potato dumplings, which always contain a small amount of flour.

Goulash. A roux-based Hungarian stew flavored with paprika.

Macaroon. A dessert cookie made of almond paste, sugar, and egg whites. Some macaroons contain a small amount of flour. Ask.

Matelote. Any fish stew made with red or white wine and thickened with flour.

Milanaise or Milanese. An Italian method of preparation usually involving veal or chicken cutlets dipped in egg and bread crumbs mixed with cheese, and fried in butter or olive oil.

Moussaka. A thick Greek eggplant casserole that is thickened with a flour-based béchamel sauce.

Navarin. A ragout or stew of mutton or lamb that has been thickened with roux.

Pasticcio. Any dish that is a mixture of meat, vegetables, or pasta and bound by eggs, béchamel sauce, and topped with bread crumbs.

Polonnaise. A popular method of preparing cauliflower involving bread crumbs.

Semolina. A fancy name for wheat flour.

Soufflé. Any sweet or savory dish that consists of pureed ingredients, thickened with egg yolks and stiffly beaten egg whites carefully folded in and baked, frozen, or refrigerated in a high-sided soufflé dish. Alas, if the based version did not contain a tiny bit of flour, it could not rise to such dizzying culinary heights, but frozen soufflés most likely do not. Ask or risk missing out on the mother of all French desserts.

Stroganoff. A ragout of beef containing sour cream, thickened with a dark roux and most commonly served over egg noodles.

And don't forget, pasta by any other name—bucatini capelli d'angelo (angel hair), cannelloni, cappellacci, cappelletti, conchiglie, fettuccine, fusilli, garganelli, lasagne, maccheroncini, maltagliatti, manfrigual, orecchiette, pappardelle, penne, pizoccheri, quadrucci, ravioli, raviolini, rigatoni, spaghetti, spaghettini, striccheti, tagliatelle, tagliolini, tonnarelli, tortelli, tortellini, tortelloni, vermicelli, ziti—is just as dangerous.

The following five terms translate into food that is safe in any language:

Fagioli. Italian for beans.

Finocchio. Not a puppet with a penchant for stretching the truth, but the Italian word for fennel, a green related to anise, but milder.

Frittata. A flat Italian omelette that is dryer than its French cousin and is never folded. It can be filled with almost anything except flour, which is never used in a frittata.

Meringue. A dessert made with egg whites and sugar. No fat. No flour.

Polenta. A white or yellow, fine-grained or coarse cornmeal that is stirred until it reaches a creamy consistency. Mixed with butter and cheese or allowed to harden, it is then fried and served as an entrée or an accompaniment. This northern Italian specialty is wheat- and gluten-free.

Restaurant Assertiveness Training Exercise

Collect your own list of foreign foods and add them to this list and learn to pronounce them properly. Make a game of finding your own favorite sauce or preparation that can be rendered wheat- and gluten-free by your favorite chef. Suggest a gratin made of your bread crumbs, a delicate batter made of rice flour, a cutlet à la Milanese using cornmeal.

Your Compliments to the Chef

Whether you have just eaten in an upscale, downscale, or medium-scale restaurant, in the neighborhood deli or a roadside diner, there is no substitute for genuine appreciation for a good meal, especially one that has been improvised just for you.

Always get up and pop your head into the kitchen to thank the chef for making something special. There is nothing better at the end of a long, bruising night behind a hot stove than the sight of a truly happy customer who has taken the time to say thanks, shake a hand, wave, blow a kiss, salute, tip a hat, tap on the kitchen window, or touch the fingers to the lips in the universal gesture of gustatory bliss to the still-busy chef. A follow-up phone call or a note of thanks will have the person eating out of your hand forever.

Remember, this is why people run restaurants—to give people like you real pleasure through food and to receive tangible proof of having succeeded.

Fast Food and Chain Reactions

Last year my husband and I and some friends drove up to the Napa Valley from Los Angeles. We were just north of the Harris Ranch, one of the all-time great places for steaks we had decided to forgo for reasons that now seem unimportant, and were surrounded by dusty, dry fields as far as the eye could see when the hunger pangs hit. By all accounts, we were in "East Nowhere," California, forty miles shy of the nearest exit. I have no idea which fast food place we pulled into. We just pulled in and ordered.

I walked up to the counter person, put on my most pathetic face, held up my bread (never even think about a long car trip without an ample supply!), and asked that it be used to assemble a grilled chicken sandwich.

I may as well have been speaking Martian. Smiles slid off freckled faces. Suspicious stares peeked out from behind the carousel of burgers. Soft-serve ice cream machines were left to drip. Youth versus experience. Guidelines versus improvisation. Before I was able to sit down to lunch, I had worked my way up the organization chart to the manager of the franchise who was the only person in that operation authorized to place my bread on their grill. I didn't feel well afterward. Who knew there was flour in chicken? (Just because it looks like plain chicken doesn't mean it is.)

The more routinized, formularized, standardized, and franchised the restaurant, the harder it will be for you to get special attention. Even the way you are greeted comes from a fat manual on operating procedure.

However, conformity can work in your favor because once you discover a menu item you can eat, you can be pretty sure (I said pretty sure, not *completely* sure) you can trust that it will be presented, prepared, packaged, boxed, bagged, and served the same way from outlet to outlet. If you have children yourself, you know this is because the average sixteen-year-old who is waiting on you cannot be expected to discover independent thought for another five or six years and those who have broken through are usually in jobs paying more than the minimum wage.

Here are just a few examples of what you can expect from the fast food culture. By no stretch of the imagination is it a complete list of all the chains littering our highways. For others in the business of roadside, sidewalk, and strip mall eating and to whom you should, before even contemplating a meal, direct all your dietary questions, see chapter 12. I hate to say it, but some of these companies will do anything to keep from disclosing their ingredients. Isn't that against the law?

BOSTON CHICKEN

The problem probably isn't the chicken. It's what on it, under it, around it, and in the side dishes that will give you a problem. I would bet money there is flour or some glutinous substance in the cheese sauce. It's so thick, you could use it to spackle a wall.

I wish I could say they have plain, roasted chicken, but I can't. I asked several times, but the company discloses ingredients only on a per-item basis via a phone call to its customer relations department:

800-365-7000. This is not convenient when you are standing in line and don't really know what to have. I'm not suggesting you do this, but I would say if enough people asked the manager to make that phone call while twenty other people waited in line, the company might get the message that it's good for business to disclose ingredients.

Burger King

Order one all-beef Whopper (the nutritional brochure says 100 percent USDA inspected beef), and hold the bun, the processed cheese, the fries (unless you know what else shares the deep fryer), the ketchup, the mustard, the mayo. By all means order the green salad, but hold the dressing, cheese, and any stray croutons that may be lurking under the lettuce leaves. Do order the beverage of your choice as long as it's water, coffee, or a soft drink, and don't forget to bring your own bread. The idea of having a shake here gives me the shakes. So much for having it "your way."

Denny's

It would be nicer to look at this menu from the point of view of a plate that is half full, rather than half empty, but that's the way this company organizes its information.

Definite no-nos around which not to build a meal: chicken-fried steak, chicken strips, clam strips, cod, fried chicken, shrimp, and taco meat all contain wheat, as do mozzarella sticks, okra, onion rings, and seasoned fries. Do not order chili and split pea soups and forgo all forms of gravy—au jus, brown, chicken, and country. Breads would seem obviously off-limits, but rice pilaf might not. Don't order it. Other than that, Mrs. Lincoln, how did you enjoy the play?

KFC

Whether you still call it Kentucky Fried Chicken or have adapted to the new, nineties "KFC," no matter how you cut it, the operative term in this chain is "fried," as in battered, as in breading. There is a movement afoot to get "clean," as in low-fat, low-sodium, non-breaded and skinless chicken on the menu in this chain, but at the moment, even the plain rotisserie chicken lists wheat flour among the "herbs and spices" in the coating. I'm rooting for those managers and franchisees who see the future, but for now, why torture yourself? You can get a salad anywhere.

McDonald's

It's not going to be such "a nice day" after all if you get stuck here. In fact, it's going to be McBoring. You might think you can get away with a McChicken patty or the chicken strips inside the fajitas, but forget it. The former contains maltodextrin; the latter unspecified food starch.

McDonald's advertises the meat in its basic hamburger, Cheeseburger, Quarter Pounder, and Quarter Pounder with Cheese as 100 percent beef with no filler. This may be all you can eat, but only *after* you remove the special sauce, ketchup, mustard, and roll. Even the mayonnaise is a McNo-No. Ditto for dressings and hash browns. Given what else goes into the deep fryer, I wouldn't try the French fries either. If you're thinking of the McLean Deluxe Beef Patty as a welcome change from heftier burgers, that may well be for other customers, but not for you. It's lighter on fat and calories, but not on maltodextrin and wheat starch. I wouldn't risk a shake, even though I must admit that I used to love them. Maybe they'll let you have some toys from the Kids Meal. Or lettuce and tomato without the dressing.

McDonald's does not break down its ingredients in terms of what's gluten-free or not. You have to call for their list and figure it out yourself.

Taco Bell

You shouldn't have to run for the border when someone mentions stopping here. The company claims its gluten-free Tostado with refried beans, lettuce, and cheese, and the Pintos and Cheese are gluten-free. Say *muchas gracias* for small favors.

The Mall Food Court

CELIAC SENTENCED TO STARVATION IN FOOD COURT!
—Imaginary Tabloid Headline

It is not only possible but entirely likely that you will go hungry in the land of plenty—the shopping mall.

Sooner or later you are going to shop till you drop. Your stomach will growl so loudly, you won't be able to hear the announcement of a one-hour sale on designer drawer organizers. It will lead you over to the food court against your will, where you will be surrounded by exotic and strange foods such as chicken-on-a-stick, gyro, sushi burgers, and potatoes stuffed with things nature never intended.

The idea is to always, always, always eat before going out to a mall and never get stuck in a situation like this. While shopping on a full stomach not only guarantees you won't starve, it also promises another little-known benefit: Any clothes you buy will get bigger, not smaller when you're not so full.

Never mind. You forgot. Now what?

If you remembered to bring two slices of bread (never, never, never go shopping again without doing this!), now is the time to get them out, head for the nearest deli or sandwich counter, and ask if it has a toaster. Most do, so even if you don't see it, ask. A toaster is not an item people proudly display. Now order a roast turkey, roast beef, or ham and cheese sandwich, or tuna or chicken or turkey salad sandwich, and don't forget to find out which mayonnaise is being used before asking for a salad. The mustard is usually in an individual packet. Read the label before you squeeze.

If you forgot your bread, go to the nearest Mexican take-out and ask if you can buy a corn tortilla, then hand it to the sandwich person at the deli counter or simply order the sandwich you want as a platter. If you're really desperate and no one understands the concept of platter, order a sandwich and, horrible as it may sound, "eat the middle." Be careful not to order anything gooey that might stick to the bread and have to be discarded. You need all the food you can get. Tell yourself this is your own fault and resolve not to do it again.

The sandwich counter may be boring, but it is the safest place for you in the average food court. Pizza is off-limits, of course, but if you're considering scraping off the top, remember the cheese is probably processed too, which also eliminates those cheese fries you love. You don't want to know what goes into the deep fryer with the plain ones, either. Most mall meals are so battered, I sometimes wonder if there's any real food underneath, and so greasy, you can get fat just standing there watching people eat.

If you're adventurous and you're comfortable eating sushi in a food court, do so, but be prepared to pass up the dipping sauce. Ditto for stir-fry and other Chinese or Japanese entrées. If you really love this stuff, carry your own bottle of wheat-free soy or tamari. Forget anything "tempura" or "teriyaki" too.

You're better off passing up the cheese on your "loaded" baked potato too. Usually it's so thick, it's got to be full of something—flour or wheat starch, wallpaper paste. If you must, ask the clerk for an ingredient list. If it's not available, order a plain potato stuffed with salsa or keep walking.

If you're good, there's always dessert. Popcorn is filling, but watch for anything that might be coated with a malt derivative. I have no idea what's in cotton candy, nor have I ever asked, because I can't imagine anyone wanting to eat it. Most food courts have ice cream and frozen yogurt stands. While some of these confections are not exactly stingy with the butter fat, others are fat-free and many are quite safe. If you really can't afford the calories, console yourself with the idea that you're in the mall to shop, not to eat.

Ice Cream and Frozen Yogurt

BASKIN-ROBBINS

Banana Nut, Banana Strawberry, Cherries Jubilee, Chewy Baby Ruth, Chocolate, Chocolate Chip, Chocolate Almond, Chocolate Fudge, Chocolate Mousse Royale, Chocolate Ribbon, Chunky Heath Bar, French Vanilla, Gold Medal Ribbon, Jamoca, Jamoca Almond Fudge, Lemon Custard, Mint Chocolate Chip, Nutty Coconut, Old

Fashioned Butter Pecan, Peach, Peanut Butter and Chocolate, Pink Bubble Gum, Pistachio Almond, Pralines 'N Cream, Pumpkin Pie, Reeses Peanut Butter, Rocky Road, Rum Raisin, 'S'Crunchous Crunch, Vanilla, Very Berry Strawberry, Winter White Chocolate, World Class Chocolate. . .

. . . and those are just the ice creams on this company's gluten-free list.

All "light," "fat-free," "reduced sugar," "Truly Free" flavors, including frozen yogurts, ices, and sherbets and Boom Choco Laka in the "Yogurt Gone Crazy" category, are said to be blissfully and sinfully gluten-free.

That adds up to 105 out of 127 flavors these people say you can eat. If there's no Baskin-Robbins in the mall or shopping area nearest you, move!

BEN & JERRY'S

You've got to like an ice cream company that makes a flavor called Cherry Garcia. These people have a reputation for being socially conscious, politically correct, charitable, user friendly, and having one of the best factory tours you could take. Obviously, any flavor with cookie or cheesecake chunks in it is off-limits. Anything with maltodextrin and other unallowables are off-limits as well. So how come Ben & Jerry's won't say which flavors are gluten-free or wheat-free? They're concerned somebody might get sick because they cannot always vouch for their extracts, which are purchased as commodities from many different sources, a buying tactic that cannot be reflected on an ingredient label.

So why can other ice cream companies say whether their ice creams are gluten-free or not? Maybe they are less fickle with their resources. Maybe not. Gives one pause.

COLUMBO YOGURT

Stick with nonfat vanilla, chocolate, or strawberry frozen yogurt. These are the only flavors a Columbo company spokesperson would guarantee as gluten-free, but more are promised in the coming months.

I was told Columbo store owners buy their toppings from various sources and the Columbo Company will not vouch for them, so do not assume they are wheat- or gluten-free. Always ask what's in them before you pour, sprinkle, roll, dice, dip, or dunk. Stay tuned for the latest dish on gluten-free flavors.

HÄAGEN-DAZS

This company, as do I, cautions you to avoid any flavor or bar using the word *cookie, cheesecake, dough, brownie,* or *burst.* Forget Caramel Cone Explosion, unless you want to have one of your own. Häagen-Dazs says its soft-serve nonfat vanilla, chocolate, and coffee frozen yogurts are gluten-free. Forget nonfat chocolate mousse and nonfat vanilla mousse soft-serve frozen yogurt.

What's left? Ice cream. The company lists plenty of flavors on the list of what's gluten-free—Belgian Chocolate Chocolate, Brandied Black Cherry, Butter Pecan, Cappuccino Commotion, Chocolate, Chocolate Chip, Chocolate Mint, Chocolate Swiss Almond, Coffee, Coffee Chip, Deep Chocolate Peanut Butter, Macadamia Brittle, Macadamia Nut, Maple Walnut, Pralines & Cream, Rum Raisin, Strawberry, Vanilla, Vanilla Chip, Vanilla Fudge, and Vanilla Swiss Almond. And of course, there's always sorbet.

TCBY

This company may call itself "the country's best yogurt," but it's not necessarily the country's best gluten-free yogurt. A company spokesperson happily informed me that all frozen yogurt flavors are gluten-free, but when I received the list of "base" ingredients, I discovered this refers only to the base and not to the flavor that is added, which includes ingredients such as "natural and artificial flavors, fudge powder, eggnog base and cheesecake base," which were not disclosed as real or flavorings. Further inspection revealed maltodextrin in the No Sugar Added Nonfat Frozen Yogurt base. Is this called "fudging" the issue? Or just sloppy work?

Moral: I would hope we could all take reputable companies at their word, but maybe that's not the case. This is, after all, a litigious society where the company and its customers often find themselves in an adversarial relationship. We have to wonder about the frequency of label production versus the reformulating of ingredients or awarding contracts to resources, and the wheat- or gluten-free status of a product must be the subject of conjecture and a company's voluntary goodwill. Why is this not simply legislated, as sodium and fat are? If my shirt is a blend, by law the label cannot say "100% cotton." Why isn't this the case with my ice cream and other ingestible products?

Until such time as this labeling problem is straightened out, give yourself a better shot at licking any potential problems by doing the following. Call your favorite ice cream company and ask about your favorite ice cream or frozen yogurt flavors specifically. Stick with those flavors that do not cause you any problems, and periodically check with the company for updates on ingredients. Do not take *no* or *maybe* for an answer. You have a right to know. That's all you can do, short of buying your own machine. It's only ice cream, not world peace.

A final word . . . If you are still feeling less than assertive about your wheat- and gluten-free restaurant experience, you can always hire your own chef and stay home or go out with a personal taster. If you're not Oprah Winfrey, this can be very expensive. I would suggest one more tactic.

Restaurant Assertiveness Training Exercise

Rent a video of *When Harry Met Sally*. Watch it six times or until you no longer see anything unusual or funny about Meg Ryan's attitude toward ordering food.

Answers to Restaurant Quiz on Page 93:

1. (c) That old saw about first impressions has never been truer. If a restaurant employee is rude on the phone, just wait till you ask for

special treatment from the kitchen. Anyway, suffering bad service in the name of fashion went out in the eighties.

2. (c) The bread may seem like the obvious culprit, but the cheese could be processed as well. Never pick your food apart or let a waiter do it for you. Not only is there a good chance you'll get some unwanted crumbs, not asking about the cheese and starting over sends the wrong message back to the kitchen. If you don't take your diet seriously, why should the restaurant?

3. (a) Shooting from the hip is never a good idea, especially when you're hungry. Understand that the waiter is simply stating the restaurant's policy. The idea is to keep the conversation going until you get past no or it becomes apparent that you are the exception to this general rule. If this doesn't work, you have my permission to skip to answer c.

4. (b) It doesn't matter how you ask, just do it, even if you think you know what a menu term means, but you're not completely sure. You'll "roux" the day you don't.

5. (c) It's so easy to go along with the crowd. Do it often enough and you'll end up resenting your friends. Lie and they'll end up resenting you. How can you ask a restaurant for special treatment if you can't ask your friends?

CHAPTER SIX

The World Is Your Rice Noodle

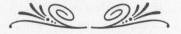

The excursion is the same when you go looking for your sorrow as when you go looking for your joy.

—EUDORA WELTY
from *The Optimist's Daughter*

If you can see beyond the basic American diet and its reliance on starchy foods, thickened gravies, bread, burgers, and deep-fried everything and develop a taste for experimenting, the world of ethnic eating can be more than your rice noodle. It can be your risotto, your enchilada, your papadum, and your pad Thai.

For years Italian restaurants were off-limits for me. The aroma of garlic and warm bread and freshly made pasta was too much. It made me feel sad and empty, as if I could never eat enough to make up for the absence of this divine and primal food. I wept at the sight of spaghetti and meatballs. I became depressed and, to the dismay of family and friends, developed the disconcerting habit of reading menus aloud, pronouncing the names of foods I could never eat, as if rolling the sound of them on my tongue was tantamount to tasting. This was not a great deal of fun for me or my dinner companions.

That was before risotto with asparagus and tre formaggio. It was before I encountered the melting warmth of polenta, stirred into a thick cornmeal mush made with fresh tomato sauce and porcini mushrooms, or in the dark days before I learned to carry my own box of pasta to all but the snootiest Italian restaurant and they would oblige me with a celiac's dream bowl of spaghetti or fettucine topped with any sauce on the menu.

Many cultures rely on rice as a staple food. Others prepare everything with corn, and still others use lentil and bean flours and other exotic and allowable ingredients. The more adventurous you are willing to become, the more you will discover how many countries do not depend on wheat- or gluten-containing grains for their cuisine.

Most notable is Mexico. As long as you remember to ask for corn tortillas to replace anything prepared with the heavier and more caloric flour version, very little on a Mexican menu is off-limits.

Many Indian dishes are made with lentil flour that has not been mixed with wheat flour. In fact, a delicious crisp Indian bread called papadum and a dish called masala dosa use lentil flour exclusively.

Thai cuisine incorporates the rice noodle into many of its dishes seasoned with the distinctive flavors of lemon grass, fiery chili oil, and coconut milk. As long as you can be assured of the absence of soy sauce, pad thai is a wonderful combination of rice noodles, shrimp, bean thread, and spices. Very few Thai restaurants do not offer this classic on their menu.

The Chinese version of this dish is usually called Singapore shrimp or Singapore noodles. If prepared well and also devoid of soy sauce, the rice noodles are a welcome change from the sticky white rice served in most Chinese restaurants.

People with grain allergies avoid ethnic restaurants unnecessarily, missing the boat on good eating because of their fear of the unknown and the unusual. As long as you are able to communicate with the chef or the waiter (if you can't, make some extra copies of the traveling cards in the appendix), the following overview on "eating ethnic" should put those fears to rest once and for all.

A note of caution. Recipes vary from restaurant to restaurant, and every chef puts his or her personal stamp on even the most traditional of dishes. As with everything you buy or order, you must always ask how a food is prepared and what's in it before you consume it. The following suggestions are merely guidelines, but they should go a long way toward helping you negotiate a menu and decide which dishes to investigate further.

Italian

If you can't see past the pizza and the pasta with tomato sauce on a typical Italian menu, you will undoubtedly go home disappointed and hungry.

Always ask for risotto. Even if it's not listed on the menu, you may find a willing chef who is grateful for the opportunity to honor such a request. More than a meal, this classic rice dish is virtually a ritual in northern Italian kitchens, and it is even more ubiquitous than pasta in Turin, Milan, and Venice, and from the Alps all the way to the Adriatic, where the best short-grained Arborio and Carnaroli rice are found. When it is prepared properly, it is rich, creamy, cheesy, savory, satisfying, and everything you miss about pasta.

Try polenta. This wonderful cornmeal dish can be served soft and mixed with cheese and any number of savory sauces, or it can be cooled and sliced, then grilled and served as an accompaniment to roasted meats and other dishes.

My idea of the perfect Italian meal is to start with a light Parma ham and melon or an antipasto plate of tuna, salami, provolone, mozzarella, prosciutto, artichoke hearts, calamari, mushrooms (make sure they are not stuffed with breadcrumbs), hearts of palm, olives, and anchovies.

Follow this with a small "pasta" portion of risotto with wild mushrooms or spring vegetables and a salad of tomatoes, fresh mozzarella, and basil with some good olive oil, a grind of pepper, and a splash of balsamic vinegar. And it doesn't get better than osso buco (veal shanks) on a bed of soft polenta for your main course (as long as the shanks have not been floured first or the brown sauce thickened with flour), unless, of course, you have ordered a veal chop accompanied by grilled polenta with sun-dried tomatoes and mushrooms or grilled tonno (tuna) marinated in olive oil, rosemary, basil, and garlic and served with broccoli di rape and rice.

If you really must have pasta, bring your own and ask that it be served with shrimp, mussels, clams, and scallops, an eggplant sauce or a spicy puttanesca sauce or placed under an order of garlicky shrimp scampi. Any safe sauce on the menu is yours for the asking with the price of a box of Pastariso or your own favorite brand of rice pasta and an affirmative response from the chef. Most Italian vegetables are done simply in olive oil and garlic, which makes them wheat- and gluten-free.

Desserts are as tough in Italian restaurants as they are everywhere else, but you never know when you are going to run into croccante, crunchy Italian pralines served with espresso or crushed over gelato, Bolognese rice cake (take care there are no bread crumbs lurking on its bottom), monte bianco, quite literally a mountain of chocolate and chestnut that has been snowcapped with whipped cream, or zabaglione, an airy concoction I have always believed to be made of Marsala wine and clouds, which are really egg yolks beaten into a froth.

If you see granita on the menu, you may not even care what is offered for dessert. This frozen Italian slush of sugar and very strong espresso, topped with whipped cream or milk, is dessert enough for any serious sweet lover. Take care the whipped cream is pure. No vanilla-flavored imitations for you.

If no such goodies appear, order your favorite gelato, a rich Italian ice cream that should be free of fillers (ask!), and always inquire how the cheesecake is made (every once in a while, you will find a light ricotta cheese cake made with no flour at all), and make sure you have your own biscotti. Buon appetito!

Japanese

If you love sushi or sashimi, you're in luck as long as you remember to bring your own wheat-free soy or tamari sauce or make sure it's provided at the restaurant. Do you remember the difference? Sushi is raw with rice. Sashimi is raw without rice. I like to order sashimi and a small bowl of brown rice when I eat Japanese. Take a little bit of the rice with a bite of the fish and it's not so filling that way. It's always good to bone up on the menu before you jump in. You never know what you might end up with otherwise. A basic course in sushi . . .

Akagai: Red clam	*Maguro*: Tuna
Amaebi: Sweet shrimp	*Mirugai*: Giant clam
Anago: Sea eel	*Saba*: Mackerel
Aoyagi: Skimmer clam	*Sawakani*: Baby octopus
Ebi: Shrimp	*Shake*: Salmon
Hamachi: Yellow Tail	*Tako*: Octopus
Hirame: Fluke	*Tamago*: Egg omelet
Hokkigai: Surf clam	*Tobiko*: Flying fish egg
Ika: Squid	*Unagi*: Clear water eel
Ikura: Salmon roe	*Uni*: Sea urchin
Katsuo: Bonito	

There are also lobster rolls, California rolls, avocado rolls, Alaska rolls, tuna rolls, crab sticks, and salmon rolls. These are rice, fish, and vegetable combinations that are often sauced. Ask first.

Tofu is soybean curd, a high-protein source that is featured prominently in Japanese cuisine and is absolutely tasteless until seasoned, fried, sautéed, or sauced. At that point it takes on the flavor of the food in which it is cooked. Always ask how tofu is done as there is a strong probability that it has been soaked or stir-fried in soy sauce.

Mozuku is seaweed served with sweet vinegar, which is invariably rice vinegar and should be safe to order if soy sauce has not been added.

Avoid anything that is described as "tempura" unless you can be sure how the batter is made. Some Japanese restaurants use rice flour for their fried dishes, so it is entirely possible your favorite is one of them. Others keep it on hand and may agree to do your order with this lighter-tasting batter. Find out before you cross this dish off your list.

Beware of soba. These buckwheat noodles often contain a mixture of buckwheat and wheat flour. If you can tolerate buckwheat, make sure that's all you're getting. Never order udon, a wheat noodle. Look for rice sticks or rice noodles and ask that they be used in your soup.

Miso is soybean broth and sumashi is clear chicken broth. Check for soy sauce before ordering these.

Gyoza is a fried beef dumpling that contains flour and soy sauce, but edamame is usually steamed soy beans with no soy sauce added.

Anything teriyaki is glazed; yakatori, glazed and skewered; and sukiyaki is a method of preparing vegetables, chicken, beef, or seafood in a soup like stew à la bouillabaisse. Order none of these. They're full of soy sauce.

There is surprisingly little wheat and gluten on Japanese dessert menus. Green tea ice cream is refreshing and often homemade, with no fillers and stabilizers, and fried bananas with honey are quite good. Yokan is not for everyone, but for those who need to know, it's sweet bean jelly.

Greek

Forget the kasseri cheese appetizer called saganaki opa! It's delicious. It's dramatic. It's flamed at the table. And it's full of bread crumbs.

Order hummus, a garlicky puree of chick peas and sesame seeds (tahini) mixed with olive oil; tzatziki, whipped yogurt with cucumbers, lemon juice, and garlic; taramosalata, whipped Greek caviar with olive oil and lemon juice; or babacunuch, a dip of roasted eggplant with garlic, oil, lemon, and tahini. These are traditionally served with pita triangles, but in your case, they are just as delicious with chilled cucumber slices. Cucumber is the mainstay of the traditional Greek peasant salad, so you shouldn't have a problem asking for a side order. If you prefer bread with your dip, toast some triangles of rice bread and take them along.

Go crazy with briny Greek olives and feta, the salty and reasonably low-fat national cheese. Dolma are grapes leaves stuffed with rice, and they are usually wheat- and gluten-free. Ask first.

Stay away from avgolemono, which is a thick Hellenic lemon and egg soup with rice and chicken broth, unless you can be positive it has been thickened with egg yolks only. Avgolemono is also served as a sauce for other Greek dishes, including the more substantial entrée of grape leaves stuffed with beef and lamb and rice, so it is important to establish its ingredients before ordering.

Pastitsio and moussaka are the Greek variations of lasagne. Both are held together with béchamel sauce, which is thickened with flour, and pastitsio usually contains a pasta called orzo. Never confuse orzo (pasta) with ouzo (a very strong drink).

While spanakopita (spinach pie) should be an obvious no-no, some Greek restaurants make a variation that is a bubbly casserole of rice, spinach, and feta cheese minus the filo dough. As with every cuisine, all thick sauces are suspect and must be explained before you order any Greek stew or braised dish.

Plaki means anything on a platter or planked and usually refers to baked or grilled fish. Grilled fish à la Greque usually involves no more than olive oil, garlic, and lemon and is as heart healthy as it is wheat- and gluten-free. Gyro is a marinated, spiced meat, sliced very thinly. I, personally, do not trust it.

Skordelia is another name for mashed potatoes so garlicky and good, you'll probably cry with happiness for having had the sense to order them. Make sure the chef did not take a short cut and use any nontraditional thickeners.

I don't miss Greek desserts because I've never really liked the overly sweet baklava and other syrupy filo dough pastries or the equally sweet galaktobouriko, a baked custard with the same potential for toothache.

I always ask about the raisin rice pudding or homemade yogurt with honey and walnuts. Once assured that these are free of thickening or vanilla, go for these more traditional and less waistline-damaging endings to a Greek meal.

Afghan

If you're like most people, you're not even sure where exactly Afghanistan *is*, much less what defines this mountain country's cuisine. I realize not every American town has a neighborhood Afghan restaurant like Philadelphia's Kabul, but for those that do, this food should be considered a stop on every wheat- and gluten-free field trip.

Unlike its neighbors, India and Pakistan, where chefs fight the fiery climates with more fire in their curries, Afghan cooking is milder, more subtle, cooler, like the temperatures at Afghanistan's higher elevation. Exotic spices and flavors predominate—cardamom, saffron, orange peel, rose water, yogurt, and mint. Lamb and yogurt feature strongly, but dishes are surprisingly mild, despite their intricate seasonings.

Skip the appetizers, which are usually turnovers, dumplings, and deep-fried pastries, and move right along to the main course. Not all restaurants use the same ingredients, so remember to ask before you consider the following.

Kabuli-palaw is a gorgeous combination of lamb, rice, carrots, raisins, almonds, and pistachios in a spiced tomato sauce. Norenge-palaw is a sweeter version of this dish with the addition of cardamom and orange peel soaked in rose water. Badenjan-chalaw combines lamb and eggplant, and facilliya-chalaw green beans and lamb.

Kabobs of chicken or lamb or ground beef are usually marinated in yogurt, spices, garlic, and lemon before cooking. In this land where meat is not as plentiful or as available as it is here, vegetables are made much of.

Buranee badenjan is sautéed eggplant with meat sauce and yogurt.

Sabzi is pureed spinach with onions, and buranee kadu is sautéed pumpkin with meat sauce and yogurt.

Afghan desserts tend to be sticky, sweet, and off-limits for the grain intolerant, but firnee,a silky Afghan pudding sprinkled with pistachios and almonds is usually thickened with cornstarch. Usually it contains no vanilla, but asking doesn't hurt.

An Afghan meal is typically finished off with green tea or chai, a traditional tea. You haven't come this far for a cup of coffee.

Middle Eastern

Bulgur wheat is a big deal in the Middle East, as in kibbie nayee, the national dish of Lebanon. And tabbouleh. Forget falafel as well.

After that, there is emjudra, a dish of lentils and rice cooked in onion broth. Many Middle Eastern restaurants serve ej-jee, a Lebanese omelet flavored with mint and onions. Hummus tahini is the Israeli and Egyptian version of mashed chick peas and crushed sesame seeds, and while babaganoush is spelled differently in Greek, it's still pureed eggplant with sesame dressing. This is a big favorite in Syria and Turkey as well.

Greek olives are called zatoon in the Middle East. Laban is said to be an authentic yogurt made from a thousand-year-old culture. I didn't think it tasted a day over five hundred. As in Greek restaurants, cucumbers abound in Middle Eastern restaurants. Ask for your own plate and enjoy the dips.

Maza is the Armenian, Turkish, and Greek answer to antipasto. Mixed dishes are always good because you can discuss their contents when you order and ask that any no-nos be left out and extras of the yes-yeses added. Another way to do this is to make a deal with your dinner partner, order two mixed plates, and rearrange to suit.

Marinades are usually yogurt, garlic, and lemon in this part of the world, but do check first before you order the kabobs.

Pass up the pastry tray and have a piece of halvah or halawah, Lebanese sugar and sesame paste candy, a glass of rose water, or maybe a nice cup of kawhwee, the dark Turkish coffee that is usually served by the thimbleful, for good reason.

Thai

The contrasts are sharp in this part of the world. Four-alarm curries, fiery chili pastes, searing peanut sauces, coconut milk, and lemon grass are the grace notes of this interesting food.

Spring rolls are often made with rice wrappers, which can be used for your own delicious purposes, as you will see in chapter 10. Bean thread or rice sticks are used in place of wheat noodles, with tofu instead of chicken or beef. Pineapple and tapioca make fried rice distinctly Thai, and lemon grass soup can lull the diner into a false sense of security, a subtle prelude to the heat of any number of Thai curries.

Pad thai is a classic dish made with rice noodles, egg, bean curd, bean sprouts, and green onion topped with ground peanuts. There are many variations on the rice noodle, as well as rice pancakes and spicy fritters of corn and potato.

The difficulty of dining safely on Thai cuisine is in the sauces. Clear fish sauce contains no wheat, but Hoisin sauce does and can affect sensitive types. Soy, tamari, and thick fish and peanut sauces are often used as well and are problems.

If you love this food, as I do, my best advice is to sit down with your local Thai chef and figure out what you can eat and what you can't together. Most Thai dishes are individually stir-fried, so it's not as if your diet is affecting the entire night's business. Naturally, you must be a good enough customer to make it worthwhile for the restaurant to clean the stir-fry pan and start over for you, and you should be considerate of peak times. You will not be sorry you took the trouble. Fresh, homemade Thai rice noodles alone are worth the effort.

Mexican

Enchiladas, tortillas, carne asada, salsa, guacamole, *carumba!* Not to mention masa harina, huevos rancheros, nachos, tostadas, and good old rice and beans. This is the land of corn and plenty and mole sauce. When a grain intolerant goes to heaven, it's usually Mexico. *A note of caution:* If you are one of those celiacs who are sensitive to chile powder, do not think of going Mexican. It's in everything. Sorry, *amigo.*

It is very important to find a good Mexican restaurant, not one of the plastic burrito factories that seem to be popping up on every major highway. The reason for this is simple. The less formularized and processed, the safer it's going to be for you. Besides, places like these are American, not Mexican.

Real Mexican cuisine uses masa harina (a cornmeal soaked in lime); tomatillos (small green tomatoes); corn husks, which are traditionally used to serve tamales; guava paste; hominy (a cereal made from corn); and flat corn bread called tortillas, which are usually homemade and bear no resemblance to the tasteless versions found in fast food stands.

Homemade salsas bear little resemblance to those watery concoctions found on supermarket shelves. Fresh ingredients and good non-processed cheddars and jack cheeses are used in everything from nachos to quesadillas, Mexico's answer to pizza. It is usually made with the larger flour tortilla but can easily be made with its smaller and gluten-free cousin. Learn to spot the difference between these two tortillas from across the room. (Hint: Corn is yellow and smaller than flour, which is white and large.) In fact, almost any dish that is made with a flour tortilla can be made with a corn tortilla. Be careful, though, that the rest of the ingredients contain no wheat or gluten. Some chefs start their chili from a roux; always ask if the chili contains any flour.

A typical Mexican menu might include gazpacho, a spicy chilled soup made of pureed tomatoes, peppers, cucumbers, and spices. Ask the waiter to leave off the croutons that sometimes accompany this dish.

Chili relleños can be made with bread crumbs or not. Make sure you know which you are ordering.

Most Mexican sauces—salsa verde, salsa rojo, salsa casera—do not contain flour. Guacamole sauce or dip is made from avocados, and mole is a spicy sauce that includes cocoa.

Beans (frijoles) are a mainstay of Mexican cuisine. Frijoles refritos (refried beans) are typically not made with any thickening, but traditionally they are fried in lard, if you're counting fat grams.

As with all cuisines, avoid any chilis, stews, or dishes that appear to be enrobed in a thick sauce. These usually contain flour. Cornstarch is used as a thickener in many Mexican recipes as a substitute for wheat flour. Always ask before you decide on a dish.

Authentic chorizos, spiced Spanish sausages used frequently in Mexican cooking, usually contain tequila, wine vinegar, and hot chilis among other spices. Never eat a chorizo whose ingredients cannot be accounted for.

The traditional Mexican dessert custard called flan usually contains vanilla. I wouldn't order it. In fact, I wouldn't recommend the dessert menu at all. Have something exotic instead, like fresh mango or guava paste, and quit while you are pleasantly full.

Spanish

While the Spanish have had an enormous influence on Mexican food, Spanish food takes its cues from the great cities of Barcelona, Valencia,

Malaga, and Granada along the Mediterranean and from the dusky sweetness of North Africa just beyond.

All over Spain, bars and bistros called *tascas* serve the tapas, or small appetizer dishes that are the national snack. Their American cousins are cropping up in cities all over the United States, where it is the custom to drink sherry, share gossip, and order from extensive menus of foods served in very small portions.

Proceed carefully. It's easy to be overwhelmed by such small portions and the speed with which they arrive at the table. In the casual, often rollicking spirit of these places, some wheat or gluten may slip by. Bypass the obvious and maybe not so obvious offenders—empadillas (turnovers), emparedos (small sandwiches), croqetas (croquettes), or any other puffs, pancakes, or balls.

Stick with simple dishes containing foods you can readily see— such as Spanish antipasto; garlic shrimp (gambas al ajillo); clams in tomato sauce (almejas al diablo); mussels marinated in red wine, capers, and pimiento (mejillones a la vinagreta); eels in garlic sauce (angulas a la bilbaina); or smelts. Order chorizo if you can ascertain how it was made. Some tapas restaurants serve miniature tortillas, which are not tortillas at all but flat Spanish omelets served in wedges. Always ask about fillings before you order. Always ask about everything.

If you are dining in a more traditional Spanish restaurant, there is always paella, the rich dish that is the centerpiece of Spanish cuisine.

There is paella à la Valenciana with chicken and seafood, paella marinera with seafood only, paella huertana de murcia with vegetables, and paella de codornices y setas, featuring quail and mushrooms. Fideua de mariscos, a paella of noodles and shellfish, is best to avoid.

Zarzuela de marisco is a spicy and spectacular shellfish stew served over rice.

Try one of the endless varieties of the hearty and filling Spanish tortillas or omelets. As with all cuisines, be wary of sauces and stews. Always ask the chef how either is thickened before ordering it.

Marzipan, the almond sugar candy, came to Spain by way of the Moors and is on many Spanish menus. In fact, so many Spanish candies are made with almonds, sugar, coconut, and eggs and no wheat or gluten, it is advisable to find a good Spanish-American market and stock up.

Skip the pastry cart and the flan, which is invariably full of vanilla, and explore baked apples, bananas with honey and pine nuts, pears in dark Spanish wine, prunes, and apricots. For once, you will not be sorry you ordered fruit.

Indian

While it is true that many Indian chefs grind their own seasonings to make curry, their magical potion, there are too few of them to consider. If you can tolerate curry, welcome to the land of vindaloo, tandoori, papadum, masala dosa, dal, raita, and mango chutney.

NOTE: Some celiacs are sensitive to commercial curry powder. If you are one of these unfortunates, skip Indian cuisine.

The basic principle of Indian cooking relies on fiery hot quenched by soothing and cool. Most dishes are usually served all at once, so the diner can decide how much of each temperature is appropriate. Desserts are deliberately mild and fragrant after a meal of such stunning contrasts.

In traditional Indian kitchens, curry is based on something called ghee, which is really butter that has been melted and skimmed of its foam several times. This ghee, or clarified butter, is the foundation for all the variations, none of which should contain flour. I say should and I will say it until it is firmly in your mind, because in an age of shortcuts, your health depends on asking each time.

Curries range from mild to very hot. Never ask for very hot unless you know what that particular chef's definition of this is. You can always ask for something a little hotter next time. If you are sweating from the top of your head or the soles of your feet, it's too late.

The vindaloo style of cooking tends to be very hot, while "tandoori" refers to the clay oven used to prepare less fiery dishes, such as chicken marinated in lemon, yogurt, garlic, and ginger.

Basmati is often the rice of choice in Indian cooking, and it is sweeter and more fragrant than the standard grain.

Raitas are the yogurt sauces that cool the hot dishes. They are usually made with cucumbers and watercress, but can be made of bananas or bananas and coconut, or eggplant or potatoes. They are always soothing and put out the fire nicely.

Bryani is an eggplant and saffron rice casserole based on ghee, and dal is a thick puree of moong (yellow split peas) or urhad dal (lentils) that is a staple food in India and one of the highest concentrations of protein you can get. Lamb and goat are familiar items on Indian menus, but vegetable dishes feature prominently as well, because so much of India's population is vegetarian for religious reasons.

Watch out for uppama. It contains farina.

Always ask what a chutney contains before trying it. Some exotic versions of this condiment contain pickled fruits and vegetables that may have spent time in vinegar and could affect those who are truly sensitive.

Khagina is an Indian omelet; akuri, scrambled eggs; aki, a poaching liquid; and pakoras, spicy vegetable fritters, usually held together with lentil flour. Never order a pakora without making sure. Ditto for dosa, a rolled rice-flour pancake filled with potatoes and spices.

Puri, chapati, nan, kulcha, roti, and paratha are all breads made of nonallowable flours. The crispy fried spiced wafers called papadum, however, are not. They are traditionally made from lentil flour. At the risk of repeating myself, ask.

Desserts in India are really unusual. Stay away from the usual suspects and experiment with rasmalai, a sweetened cottage cheese dumpling served with thickened milk, or gulab jamun, cardamom- and saffron-spiced balls of milk curd in sugar syrup served hot.

There's always Darjeeling tea or the spicy minted variety called masala, but you really can't call yourself experimental until you've tasted masala lassi, a traditional spiked buttermilk drink, or mango lassi, a wonderful yogurt drink with mango.

Chinese

As with Mexican food, find a really good Chinese restaurant. Much of what is found in the average Chinese take-out is just that, average. It is also loaded with soy sauce and MSG.

In order to enjoy good Chinese cooking, you need to get on speaking terms with the chef. Since many Chinese chefs do not speak English well or at all and Mandarin isn't exactly a second language in most American neighborhoods, you may want to use your traveling card. (See appendix.) Do whatever it takes to get a good Chinese meal on the table.

Chinese cooking uses an enormous amount of soy sauce and other sauces that contain it. I love rice noodles (bi fun), especially stir-fried with shrimp and pork curry or with vegetables, but they can't be ordered in just any Chinese restaurant. Nor can you order guon fun, rice roll with vegetables and meat. You must make sure the chef has adapted it for you or prepare it yourself with wheat-free soy sauce.

As a rule, Chinese chefs thicken with cornstarch. Pass up pickled items. Many items are imported from China, and it's virtually impossible to know what's in the pickling mixture.

Before you give up on China, look for chrysanthemum soup, a light chicken soup afloat in chrysanthemum petals, or one of the egg drop, egg curd, or ginger broth varieties, which should be free of soy sauce. Forget the Szechwan favorite, hot and sour. It's always made with soy sauce.

Keep an eye out for the exotic tea eggs, which are made with star anise, black tea leaves, cinnamon, and preserved ginger or preserved ancient eggs, traditionally made with duck eggs, lime, black tea, and fireplace ashes. Peking stirred eggs, the Chinese version of ham and eggs, are wonderful and usually do not contain soy sauce.

Peking duck, with its deep mahogany lacquer of honey, is gorgeous when prepared properly. This dish can be made with molasses as well. Make sure you know the difference, if you don't tolerate molasses well, and forgo the plum sauce unless you know what's in it. Pass up the Hoisin sauce entirely. Tea-smoked duck is also very good and should not be prepared with anything but spiced salt, lemon or orange, rice, brown sugar, and black tea leaves. Remember what I said about the sauce. Any sauce.

Dim sum is Chinese for "dough."

Read your fortune before passing the cookie to someone else. It should say, "Confucius say, have the dragon eye pudding for dessert." This Shanghai classic is usually made with rice flour. It wouldn't be as much fun if I told you what longans, or dragon's eyes, are.

Brazilian

This is barbecue country. There is no place to hide wheat or gluten in a steak that comes straight from Brazil's ranches or from the pampas of its neighbor, Argentina. If you like good beef, this is the country of origin.

If not, bacalhau is dried, salted codfish and very popular in Brazil. Acaraje are black-eyed pea fritters, which should be made from pure black-eyed pea flour.

Seviche is popular all over South and Central America. Whether it is shrimp, scallops, lobster, octopus, bass, or black conch, it is always raw fish that has been marinated in fresh lime or the juice of Seville oranges and peppers, tomatoes, chilis, onion, and other ingredients for at least six hours. The fish loses its translucence and fishy taste in the juice and needs no further cooking. Really.

Quibe is winter squash soup or, sometimes, West Indian pumpkin, but it does not require thickening except vegetable puree. A true Bahian shrimp stew does not contain flour.

A good Brazilian restaurant will prepare salt cod (bacalhau) many ways: in chili and almond sauce or Bahia style with coconut milk and tomato, a Mineira with cabbage, or with eggs.

Roupa Velha means "old clothes" in Portuguese. It is also the name for a stew of shredded or leftover flank steak. Before you order it, ask the chef if it has been thickened with flour.

Feijoada completa is the national dish of Brazil. The recipe can include everything from dried salt pork; salted beef; pig's ears, tail, and feet; tongue; pork sausage; kielbasa; Brazilian sausage (linguica); and turtle beans. A major discussion is in order before you attempt to order this. There are too many variables here.

Brazilian chocolate mousse is usually made with cashews, and coconut blanc mange is typically thickened with anything but cornstarch. Remember, this is America, land of shortcuts. Ask the chef, anyway.

Cha is tea, and Guarana is Brazil's favorite soft drink.

Scandinavian

It's very cold in this part of the world, and there is quite a bit of fish, especially codfish. For this reason, you will find quite a bit of pickled and salted food. This means vinegar, which you must be very careful to avoid in a Danish, Swedish, Norwegian, or Finnish restaurant, especially on a smorgasbord, the traditional Scandinavian buffet table.

Moving beyond the stereotype, you should find Danish hot buttermilk soup, apple soup, cherry soup (kirsebaersuppe), and summer vegetable soup thickened with nothing but cornstarch. Swedish meatballs usually contain bread crumbs. You won't know until you ask. If you have to ask about beer soup, you should not be allowed to go out for dinner.

Gravad lax is Swedish marinated salmon, and it's worth the price of admission.

You will find reindeer, whale, and venison on menus in Scandinavian countries, and you may find these meats in Scandinavian-American restaurants. If you do and can handle it—I draw the line at Rudolph—don't get so caught up in your ability to try new things that you forget to ask how they are prepared.

Danish ham is a real treat. Watch for mustard and bread crumbs in the coating and Madeira sauce in the glaze. Madeira is based on a brown stock that can, in turn, be based on a roux, or flour paste.

As in all restaurants of the world, watch out for sauces. The lands of the midnight sun love to put vinegar in theirs.

Norwegian prune pudding, which is traditionally thickened with cornstarch, and Swedish rice porridge, a traditional Christmas dessert, should not contain vanilla; Danish prune custard does.

Akvavit, the traditional fire water of Scandinavia, is usually made from potatoes. All too often it isn't. Sorry.

African

In Swahili, *karamu* is the word for "feast." Unusual flavors come together in Africa because of the vast differences in climate, temperatures, and confluence of cultures. North African cuisine is heavily grain based and therefore difficult, featuring couscous and teff, an Ethiopian grain. Curries abound and further complicate life for those who cannot tolerate these seasonings. I would book a table elsewhere on the continent.

Papaya and chile soup is a South African specialty mixing two unexpected flavors. Traditionally cornstarch is used as a thickener.

Tanzanian fruit and cashew salad with rum cream is worth searching for, and so is the beef and plantain cake from Kenya called matoke. Not a real cake, this is a casserole of highly spiced pieces of beef that have been folded into a plantain and spinach puree, then baked and garnished with shredded coconut.

Cachupa is an exotic vegetable stew of kale, corn, lima and kidney beans, bananas, name (white yam), and calabaza (acorn squash), among other exotic ingredients from the Cape Verde Islands off the coast of West Africa. This traditional dish often contains chorizo (Spanish sausage), and it's important to find out how that is made before ordering.

Beware of bobotie. This curried beef casserole from South Africa contains bread crumbs.

Yassa is a spicy marinated chicken in onion sauce from Senegal that can be served over rice or couscous. Find out which one is used in your restaurant, then ask that yours be served over rice.

Doro wat is an Ethiopian chicken stew that should not be made with any wheat or gluten. It is typically served over injera, a flat bread made of teff, which is not allowed. Order this over rice and explain why, so as not to be perceived as rude or unconcerned about tradition.

Angolan shrimp are marinated in a spicy mixture that may turn up on the menu as piri-piri, pilli-pilli, or even peri-peri. There should be no wheat or gluten in any of these versions.

Tiebou dienne are Senegalese fish filets stuffed with rice. If prepared properly, they should not contain bread crumbs.

Pass up kotokyim, the crab gratin from Ghana. Like gratins everywhere, this one contains bread crumbs.

Drink a cup of strong coffee, soothing mint tea. Then make a *tamshi la tutaonana* (farewell statement) in Swahili or just say thank you and pay your bill.

Caribbean

The flavors of Africa, Spain, France, and other European colonists predominate and mix with the island abundance of fresh fish and fruit, resulting in a few special dishes worth noting.

Ginger beer is not real beer. This West African import is made with fresh ginger, honey, and lemon. No malt. Sorrel tea is also a wonderful ginger-based refreshment from Jamaica.

Fried plantains are a Caribbean staple. Just make sure they are not breaded and, if possible, find out what else is fried in the pan or deep fryer.

For years I would not order an odd-sounding dish called fungee or fungi, which is also called coo coo or cou cou, depending on whether you are in Trinidad, Antigua, or Barbados. This is really the Caribbean answer to polenta. Jug jug is the Barbadian version with chicken and peas. But be careful of this one. It could contain millet; while it is wheat-free, it is not free of gluten.

The Conquistadores gave the Caribbean a dish called Cristiaos y Moros (Christians and Moors), which refers to the white rice and black beans that give it its stunning appearance.

There is always good fish on a Caribbean menu. The highly spiced "jerk" style of cooking refers to the distinctive Caribbean paste of scallion, chili, and allspice that is rubbed into the flesh before slow cooking over coals. It is wonderful, but don't order it unless you can determine the ingredients of the marinade.

Stay away from stews unless you can be positive they do not contain flour as thickening.

Russian

With apologies to Boris Yeltzin, who also likes the title *Against the Grain*, Russia is not a great place for people who cannot tolerate wheat or gluten.

Siberia seems to be the dumpling and noodle capital of the world with pelmeni, vereniki, haluski, and manti. With breads and savories such as kulebiaka, khachapuri, pirozhki and pirogs, Russian stroganoffs, Ukranian crepes, blini, and all the thick cabbage and beet dishes of the Baltics, you may ask yourself what's left. Plentski.

Georgian rice and lamb pilafs are fragrant and filling and are made with nuts and candied orange peel. One in particular, from Azerbaijan, can be made with an egg, potato, pumpkin, or bread crust. Make sure you know which one is being used. Or better, ask that yours be prepared with egg, pumpkin, or potato.

Borscht or kolodniy is always good. Just make sure the vinegar in it is apple cider, not white.

Say *nyet* to tabbouleh. This bulgur wheat is often prepared as a pilaf. Always make sure the one you are ordering is made with rice.

Have a Russian omelet with sour cream and caviar. Or stuffed prunes. Lamb stew with chestnuts and pomegranates is a traditional Azerbaijani dish that should not contain flour as a thickener, but as always, you must ask.

Every country has its version of polenta, and Moldavian cornmeal mush is really very good.

Kasha and wild mushroom casserole sticks to the ribs for the wheat-free and those celiacs who can tolerate buckwheat groats.

Rice-stuffed grape leaves are Russian, as are stuffed apples, quinces, peppers, and pumpkins. Lamb is often used for stuffing as well. These dishes should not contain bread crumbs or any flour thickener, but do check with the kitchen.

Mashkitchiri is literally mashed mung beans, vegetables, and rice.

Watch out for kabobs. They are often marinated in vinegar before they are cooked.

Forget dessert. Have some halvah with a glass of tea.

German

German food isn't just hard to swallow on a wheat- and gluten-free diet, it's the "wurst." There's bierwurst, bratwurst, blutwurst, bockwurst, knackwurst, leberwurst, mettwurst, weisswurst, zungenwurst, and just plain wurst—approximately 1,500 kinds of sausages, or wursts, all containing who knows what. It doesn't get any better.

There's bier. A different kind for every man, woman, and stein in Germany.

After that, there are spaetzle and schnitzels, weiner and holsteiner among them. There are dozens of brotes (breads), including pumpernickel, and there is sauerbraten, pfeffernusse, pfannkuchen, pastete, nudeln, nockerl, knodel, kuchen, kasekuchen, lebkuchen, baumkuchen, elisenlebkuchen, and gulasch. Never mind what all these words mean. To you, it's German for "you can't order it."

Not everything is verboten—you can have cabbage or potatoes, for example, as long as they're not swimming in cream sauce or crust. It's just that all the really good German dishes are loaded with flour or bread crumbs or beer or something that will arouse feeling of deprivation right down to your liederhosen.

Have some strawberries mit schlag, which is whipped cream. Or maybe just a slice of muenster and a glass of wasser while you're thinking of where else to go that won't make you cry.

CHAPTER SEVEN

Have Allergy, Will Travel

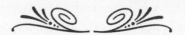

> *. . . wherever you go for the rest of your life, it stays with you,*
> *for Paris is a moveable feast.*
>
> —ERNEST HEMINGWAY
> from *A Moveable Feast*

"*Pardon, monsieur. Je ne mange pas mon pied.* Why is the waiter looking at me like that?"

"He's looking at you like that because you just said, 'Pardon me, sir. I can't eat my foot.'"

I think I hold the record for the most beginner classes ever taken at the Alliance Francaise. Like anyone who was brought up in the salsa pot that is New York City, I studied Spanish in school, while the more popular "Spanglish" peppered my conversation in the street. I did not discover the lyrical cadences of French until the window of opportunity slammed shut on that part of my brain that holds the ability to absorb new language patterns.

To further complicate my getting a firm grasp on the basics, I held a fairly senior creative position in an advertising agency, which means at one point during each semester, I was required to manage one crisis or another, lock myself in a room with other overtired writers and art directors, come up with an idea that would win a new account or keep an old one happy for at least another quarter, and fall hopelessly behind in my studies.

At the usual point in my third round of French 101, I phoned my regrets and like poor Sisyphus doomed to push that boulder up the hill once more, resolved to begin again. *"Je m'appelle Jax. J'habite a Philadelphie . . ."* My teacher suggested I start with their intermediate class next time and make up the rest of the basics on my own. *Mais non!* I would do it until I got it right.

A smattering of words in any language is usually enough to navigate a foreign city and can be considered quite charming to the locals who only fault those Americans who do not try at all, but insist on shouting English louder and louder as if addressing a crowd of deaf mutes. While I certainly considered my limitation with French an embarrassment, I had never considered it dangerous until my sprue was diagnosed and I found myself on a plane to the toughest city in the world for a celiac.

Suddenly France became one long baguette. The French word for bread and its English meaning were not lost on me. Paris had become "the city of pain," an endless tray of patisserie. The irony of having descended from people called Petitpain on my mother's Gallic side was impossibly cruel. Imagine a person called "littlebread" who is unable to eat the stuff. *Quelle horreur!*

I did not trust my grasp of French enough to buy a pair of shoes, much less to explain such an important eating problem, and I did not want to miss one bite of anything I could eat safely. So with the help of my primer, pages curling from peeking at the answers in the back, I hit upon the brilliant idea of using my rudimentary grasp of the language to explain my problem *"en francais,"* figuring this would keep me from losing my head as well as my command of the language and asking that no gloves be put into my food.

I wrote up a little card, which is probably in tatters now, somewhere in the bottomless maze of drawers and boxes that house my mementos. Nevertheless, it said in the most stilted and ridiculous school-girl French, "Please, monsieur, I must be excused from the eating of grain as my stomach will become an illness in your restaurant."

One look at my hopeless plea for help and the snootiest waiters in Paris softened in the presence of this poor soul who couldn't eat patisserie or write a simple French sentence. The manager of a little place called Le Petit Zinc pressed a bottle of Brouilly into my bag and would not roll the pastry cart to my table, shaking his head at my husband as if to say "If you ask me to do this for you, you are a cruel man." Another waiter read my card and served me nothing but cheese and vegetables. I had no idea how to ask him if flour was involved in the making of the cheese molds, so I simply said, *"Merci."* One lovely spring evening in a sidewalk restaurant in the shadow of St. Sulpice, a party broke out because of my *"petite carte."*

I had given it to the manager of that bustling café when we were seated and we had tucked ourselves up to the table, he had begun to laugh (by this time I had gotten used to this reaction to my pitiful message) and asked if he could keep it. When I said no, he gestured wildly, pressed it to his heart, and showed it to a table full of regulars who were dying to know why their friend was laughing at the American woman. One by one they peered at the card, passed it around, and, each in turn, looked over at us and waved, as intent on my husband as they were on the woman who could *"ne mange pas farin."*

Finally one of them approached our table, a jovial Brit who explained that my husband, who is also English and sports an impressive handlebar mustache, looked exactly like "Capitaine Haddock," a blustery English naval officer in the popular French cartoon strip, "Tintin." I reminded them of the hapless princess locked in the tower or, in my case, a pastry shop.

Now that we were in on the joke, tables were joined, introductions made, my card returned, and, amid the clatter of waiters, small yapping dogs leashed to the legs of tables, tourists, young lovers, gypsies, and a gnarled old couple who were moved to waltz to music drifting down to the street from an open window somewhere, a memorable and wheat- and gluten-free time was had by all.

Forget going it alone. Just match the translations in the appendix—one for wheat allergies and a longer version for celiac sprue—with the country you're visiting, photocopy them, and use them not only to order food in restaurants, hotels, sidewalk cafés, food markets, and on trains, but to strike up a conversation or spark an adventure, knock down the walls that always surround the stranger. And remember, laughter doesn't always mean someone is making fun of you. Lift your palms, raise your shoulders, roll your eyes, and smile. Like Tennessee Williams's Blanche Dubois, "Rely on the kindness of strangers." Remember, a stranger is only a friend you haven't met yet.

Worried about losing points for looking like a tourist? Worry more about eating like one or, worse, spending your entire vacation in various bathrooms, where you might consider penning the ultimate coffeetable book—*The Compleat Guide to Loos, Toilets, W.C.'s, Pottys, Privvys, Chamber Pots, Commodes, and Outhouses Around the World.*

If you must worry about something, worry about something important, such as how the dollar is doing against the pound or the Deutsch Mark or the kwatcha or the yen, or whether to hire a driver for the Amalfi coast or risk sudden death and drive it yourself. Worry about whether you've packed enough galoshes for your tour of the Lake District where, lucky for you, celiac disease and wheat allergy are commonly understood, English is spoken, and Scottish salmon is blissfully free of any offending grain.

Before you leave home, I strongly advise making several photocopies of the appropriate translation for your suitcase, suit pockets, fanny pack, passport case, wallet, and the like. Don't forget to tuck one in the evening bag and the suit pocket you're packing for the Big Night Out, and make a few extra copies for the inevitable request for a souvenir. Long after you're gone, they will speak of your visit as "The Night of the Curious American Who Could Not Eat Wheat or Grain."

You will be amazed at how many people ask to keep your card. If I am staying in a hotel for any extended period of time, I jot my room number on it and give it to the restaurant and to the room service manager. It's also a great place to scribble a note of thanks, an address, and a request for the wheat- or gluten-free recipe. A word of caution and a small disclaimer here: A translation is only as good as the understanding of it. Though I wish I could, I cannot vouch for the literacy or the intelligence of the people who may read your cards and prepare your meals. The idea is to ask for help, not to abdicate responsibility.

Have a lovely time and do drop me a postcard. I adore feedback, especially from exotic places.

Bon voyage!

Training Exercise

Don't even think about calling a railroad for information on food for short trips (several hours). It's really not worth it unless you have to be on board overnight. I'd rather starve than listen to traveling music and irritatingly pleasant voices telling me the world is just outside my window and would I please hold for another two or three hours until a real person is located. You could miss a meal just waiting to find out what's for lunch. Most trains have café cars, and sandwiches and snacks are the same the world over. Eat before you leave, pack something to nibble en route, and have something when you get where you're going. If you don't, you'll regret it.

Amtrak (800) 233-6633

Sorry, railroad buffs. With some advance notice and, of course, reservations, Amtrak will make available vegetarian, kosher, salt- and sugar-free menus, and, as of May 1, 1995, they've even designated some long-distance, overnight trains smoke-free so travelers who don't enjoy dining in a rolling ashtray can do so unmolested. When I called, they had never heard of gluten, much less given any thought to providing a meal free of it. No wheat-free menu, either. This is fine for short hops, but I would have my reservations about seeing the United States this way. It's a great view, but you can't eat it. Better get over your fear of flying.

Rail Canada (514) 871-1331

Wheat and gluten intolerance is a much bigger problem in Canada than in the United States. This is good news for you and your lifelong desire to cruise through the Canadian Rockies and visit Lake Louise, Vancouver, Jasper, Edmonton, and Alberta. With a confirmed reservation and a week's notice for all overnight excursions, the chef will be happy to prepare wheat- and gluten-free meals for you in the dining car.

Europe simply isn't that big, and most rail trips are not overnight and do not include meals. However, for those that do and for longer excursions and rail tours of exotic places, such as India, China, and South America, I would suggest booking directly through Eurail, one of the more reputable tour companies, or your own trusted travel agent. This way you will be able to make your request well in advance of your departure, in English and preferably in writing. Despite this, something can go wrong and usually does.

Many years ago, two friends who can and do eat grain missed their vaporetto and the last train to anywhere in Italy and were forced to sleep in the station with nothing but a shuttered spaghetti shop to sharpen their appetites. By morning they were ravenous. The vendor opened for business minutes before their train arrived and by the time they realized he had given them no utensils, the train was moving and they were faced with eating spaghetti with their fingers or starving. Always carry food on foreign trains, and do the other passengers a favor: Carry utensils. Anything can happen.

There is, of course, one notable and very grand exception. Grain intolerants go on honeymoons too.

THE VENICE-SIMPLON ORIENT EXPRESS (800) 524-2420

Booked through Abercrombie & Kent Tours, this is the Hercule Poirot of trains, thoroughly elegant, quintessentially European, and extremely expensive. The food is stunning. With no less than two weeks' notice, which shouldn't cause any undue inconvenience (one doesn't simply "hop" on the Orient Express), the company assures us the chef can and will handle most special diets. A trip like this should not disappoint you on any level, and I don't think it's enough simply to request a special meal, then sit back and wait to see what is served. I am told the menu changes every four months. Why not ask that it be sent to you as soon as it is available, then study it and come up with specific questions, perhaps even a suggestion or two on how it can be tailored to your diet, so this trip is the culinary delight it should be. This is once in a lifetime, *n'est-ce pas?*

You will find telephone numbers for six other foreign rail services in the Resources chapter, page 248).

Plane-ing Ahead

Contrary to what the advertising would have you believe, the skies are not friendly to people who have not ordered their meals in advance. Recently I traveled to Florida for a family emergency with no time to order a gluten-free meal. The dinner served was lasagne and a cookie. I begged the flight attendant to look for any extra special meals that had not been claimed—vegetarian, diabetic, fruit plate, salt-free, fat-free, cruelty-free, I didn't care. He told me I was in luck and said he would deliver a kosher meal after the others were served. I offered my lasagne to the man next to me who had staked a visual claim on it the second he heard my request. As he greedily consumed my dinner, I waited.

I had no idea couscous was kosher.

With time on my hands while everyone was eating, I drew a cartoon in which the passenger wore rubber gloves to accept her dinner tray and wondered aloud how many food groups were represented in a Peppermint Patty.

The definition of what is and what isn't a gluten-free meal differs from airline to airline, and unhappily too many carriers define it as any food served with a rice cake. In September 1994, on connecting flights from Philadelphia to San Diego, USAir defined my preordered gluten-free meals as requiring seven-grain crackers and a vinegar, food-starch, and maltodextrin-laden salad dressing. That's a long ride when you're hungry, queasy, and angry.

Reservation requirements vary as well; some companies require as much as a three-day notice and others as little as six hours. Most cannot confirm what will be served on your flight, but if you ask, they will give you the details of a meal that "might" be served. With rare exception, airlines do not distinguish between wheat-free and gluten-free meals, so I would recommend ordering gluten-free for the truly sensitive wheat allergic, rather than taking a chance on the regular fare. Of course, you can always order a fruit plate. Some are quite good, but that's not the point, is it?

For the most part, the skies are not appetizing for people like us. With so many fine wheat- and gluten-free products on the market, I hope that someday we will see gluten-free meals that include breads and cakes and cookies made with allowable flours, and that some clever airline marketing person figures out where I get my wheat- and gluten-free goodies and gives that company a big fat catering contract. It's a competitive world out there and, given my druthers, I'd certainly rather spend my air miles with the smart company that served gluten-free bagels and biscotti.

Until then, fasten your seat belt and butter your rice cake.

AER LINGUS (800) 223-6537

While Aer Lingus appreciates at least twenty-four hours' notice for special meal requests, it asks that you give at least three days' notice in order to insure that special gluten-free foods are on your flight. (The company says it needs the time to guarantee delivery of these hard-to-find foods.) No specifics, but I get the feeling these people are going to give you more than a rice cake.

AIR CANADA (800) 776-3000

Gluten-free meals are served with twenty-four hours' notice. There is the breakfast omelet; at dinner the possibility of poached salmon, filet of salmon, or chicken breast with tarragon; for lunch, the award goes to Air Canada for most interesting use of two rice cakes— the chicken sandwich!

AIR FRANCE (800) 237-2447
Non.

AIR INDIA (800) 223-7776

While no specifics are available, the company assures the traveler that any special meals will be made available with forty-eight hours' notice at no additional charge. My advice is that when you make your reservation, request papadum, that wonderfully crisp Indian bread made with lentil flour.

AIR JAMAICA (800) 523-5585

Gluten-free meals are available. It is suggested that you state your request very clearly, as in "I need a special gluten-free meal" an entire week ahead of time.

AIR NEW ZEALAND (800) 262-1234

With seventy-two hours' notice, this airline will serve you a gluten-free meal that contains no wheat, barley, rye, or oats, according to the brochure. As New Zealand is a long way to go when you're hungry, I'd write for it and be prepared for this long flight.

ALASKA AIRLINES (800) 426-0333

Sorry. You'll have to get to the glacier without a gluten-free meal. The management recommends the fruit plate.

ALITALIA (800) 223-5730

This Italian airline will serve gluten-free with a week's notice, but will not specify what the meal is.

AMERICAN AIRLINES (800) 433-7300

With a minimum notice of six hours, gluten-free meals are available on all domestic and international flights. A typical breakfast includes fresh fruit, scrambled eggs, potatoes, jam, margarine, and an apple cinnamon rice cake. Lunch and/or dinner can be grilled chicken with salsa or green beans, grilled zucchini or salad with gluten-free dressing, fresh fruit, and another apple cinnamon rice cake.

AVIANCA (800) 284-2622

With twenty-four hours' lead time, this airline promises to supply "absolutely anything you want."

BRITISH AIRWAYS (800) 247-9297

This is the way you want to fly wheat- or gluten-free. With at least twenty-four hours' notice, you can have either type of meal on all flights, including the Concorde, which includes five courses at the same high standard as regular meal service. There are rice cakes for breakfast with fresh fruit, scrambled eggs, and grilled mushrooms and tomatoes. Lunch may be poached salmon or smoked duck, gluten-free bread, and cheese. A snack may net you prawn egg and watercress sandwiches on gluten-free bread, gluten-free chocolate or ginger biscuits or carrot cake, and a sample dinner appetizer is smoked salmon on gluten-free toast.

CHINA AIRLINES (800) 227-5118

Forty-eight hours' notice will get you a gluten-free meal, and a spokesperson said gluten-free Melba toast, sweets, snacks, cakes, and cookies are served. I would check closer to departure time for specifics.

CONTINENTAL AIRLINES (800) 525-0280

No-salt, low-fat, diabetic, Hindu, kosher, vegetarian, semivegetarian, and fish-only meals are available. No gluten-free.

DELTA (No toll-free number; use local city number)

Six hours is all that is required to reserve a domestic or an international gluten-free meal. Breakfast might be strawberries, honeydew, canteloupe, scrambled eggs or an omelet, and potatoes served one of several ways. Lunch and dinner might be chef salad, cold cuts, spinach salad, grilled swordfish, chicken, or steak. Everything comes with a rice cake. A warning—there is no food to speak of on Delta's business express. Carry a snack in your briefcase.

EL AL ISRAEL AIRLINES (800) 223-6700

Representatives say "gluten-free meals are available, but very difficult." When asked what special gluten-free foods were served, I was told there was gluten-free bread available, but that it isn't always served. "If the other passengers get it, you'll get it. If they don't, you don't." Well, I guess they told me! Not willing to criticize an entire airline for two employees, I called again. This time I was told that "basically, a gluten-free meal on El Al is what everybody else gets stripped of the gluten." *Oy.*

FINNAIR (800) 950-5000

Gluten-free meals cannot be guaranteed with less than forty-eight hours' notice. Rice cakes are always available, I'm told, but the rice almond bread is hard to get. Maybe I should tell them where I get mine?

IBERIA AIRLINES OF SPAIN (800) 772-4642

Gluten-free meals are available with at least twenty-four hours' notice, and more is really preferred. No sample menus are available, but supposedly all package labels will be provided to the passenger and no processed food without a label or ready access to the ingredients will be used. All breads and starches are made with arrowroot, corn, potato, or rice starch. Nothing is breaded, no condiments that may contain hydrolyzed protein are used, and breakfast cereals are either rice or corn. The gluten-free bread mix contains corn, potato, rice, and/or soybean flour, and corn tortillas and rice cakes are available. *Muchas gracias!*

Japan Airlines (800) 525-3663

Gluten-free meals are available with at least forty-eight hours' notice. If you carry your own wheat-free soy or tamari, you will be able to use it only in first class, where sushi appetizers are served. JAL's computer says a roll is not necessary with this meal, which is the same as standard fare except for that. Bottom line: This airline is gluten-free by elimination, not by substitution.

KLM Royal Dutch Airlines (800) 374-7747

Gluten- and wheat-free meals are available as of March 27, 1994. No sample meals are available because the chef creates gluten- and wheat-free menus for each city KLM departs. Believe it or not, I was given the names of the North American catering manager and his assistant, who told me to have the agent call when I knew which city I was departing from, personally assuring me that any special gluten-free requests would be on board for me. All of this with no idea I was researching this book. This airline doesn't simply offer good service, it has raised it to a new standard. People like this deserve as much notice as humanly possible to help them deliver this extraordinary service.

Korean Air (800) 438-5000

Gluten-free meals are available with forty-eight hours' notice. No specific meals could be described, but products containing starches made from arrowroot, corn, rice starch, rice, and soybean flour are used in place of wheat-based foods. Corn tortillas and rice cakes are also available.

LAN CHILE AIRLINES (800) 488-0070

No gluten-free meals are available. The representative assured me that the airline would order something special to accompany a specific reservation, but his lack of understanding of what gluten- and wheat-free meals consist of did not build confidence. Pack some homemade sandwiches, gluten-free cookies, fresh fruit, and a nice big bottle of mineral water.

LUFTHANSA GERMAN AIRLINES (800) 645-3880

Gluten-free meals are available with twenty-four hours' notice. A review of a sample menu revealed a breast of "young" chicken (does anyone serve "old" chicken?), beef medallions, and a nice-sounding cold lunch of seafood salad, sliced veal, or turkey or chicken. Even better, rice or cornbreads are served in place of wheat breads on all flights. *Ich bin ein Berliner.*

MEXICANA AIRLINES (800) 531-7921

No gluten-free meals are officially served and no enchiladas are served in flight, but the crew will be happy to heat up a corn tortilla for you.

MIDWEST EXPRESS AIRLINES (800) 452-2022

Gluten-free meals are available with twenty-four hours' notice, but when the representative suggests a fruit plate . . . enough said.

NORTHWEST AIRLINES (800) 225-2525

Whether you travel domestically or internationally, twelve hours' notice will get your gluten-free meal on board. When you peel off the foil, you will see standard eggs, any style, orange juice, baked tomato, salad, rice or baked potato, red meat, or seafood without breading and with gravy made from cornstarch, plus fresh fruit and Jell-O. The rice cake comes with the fruit and cheese snack.

QANTAS (800) 227-4500

I was told via personal letter from the America's customer relations manager that I could request a gluten-free meal, ideally with twenty-four or more hours' notice, but that one would be available up to six hours prior to departure. While no sample meals could be given, I was assured that every gluten-free meal that goes "down under" does so without wheat, rye, oats, and barley or foods made of these, including luncheon meats, meat substitutes, malt products, thickened sauces, and confectionary and does include fresh fruits, vegetables, fish, chicken, milk, cheese, yogurt, and gluten-free cereal foods.

Sabena Belgian World Airlines (800) 955-2000

Gluten-free meals are available on forty-eight hours' notice, and no sample meals would be given out. Gluten-free waffles? Don't count on it.

Scandinavian Airlines (800) 221-2350

Gluten-free meals are available with at least, and *at least* is emphasized, twenty-four hours' notice. No other information regarding the exact nature of the food would be given out. I'm guessing salted fish.

Singapore Airlines (800) 742-3333

Here you'll get no wheat, oats, or barley with three days' notice.

Swissair (800) 221-4750

Gluten-free meals are available with at least forty-eight hours' notice, and no sample meals are available. With Swiss precision, I was told all gluten-free meals are made with low-fat dairy products; fresh fish, salads, and fruits; low-fat fish; lean meats; rice; and gluten-free biscuits. No sausages, pasta, custards, pastries, cakes, or chocolate will be served. I begged them to take chocolate off the no-no list.

TAP Portugal Airlines (800) 221-7370

With forty-eight hours' notice, you may order a gluten-free meal, but no details will be revealed without a confirmed reservation.

TWA (800) 221-2000

No gluten-free meals are available and no regular meals could be confirmed as gluten-free at this writing, except the fruit platter, nor could the fish be confirmed as broiled, poached, or breaded. Best bets—take the airline's advice and order the fruit plate and carry your own cheese and crackers. Or take mine—fly with people who are more considerate.

United Airlines (800) 241-6522

All gluten-free meals on United Airlines are made with meat, poultry, fresh fish, rice, eggs, fresh fruits, eggs, corn, sweet pepper, herbs and spices, potatoes, aged cheese, dairy products, yogurt, chocolate, sugar, preserves, margarine, vegetables, dried beans and peas, and nothing else. In other words, nothing special, such as rice cakes, will be served. With forty-eight hours' notice, the above items will be rearranged into a meal.

USAir (800) 428-4322

Gluten-free meals are available on twenty-four hours' notice. The representative states, "No meal containing grains or semimanufactured products containing small amounts of flour will be served." There is scrambled eggs and ham steak for breakfast; filet mignon, rice, and veggies for dinner; fruit plate, nuts, and dried fruits for snacks; and your basic rice cake, which qualifies everything as gluten-free.

Varig Brazilian Airlines (800) 468-2744

Gluten-free meals are available with at least twenty-four hours' notice, and it is requested that you give more, as this airline prepares its own food. No sample menus are available, but I am told "no processed or canned foods, nothing high in fat, only lean meats, fresh poultry and seafood; no lamb or pork, only fresh fruits and vegetables; no canned anything is used. Cornbread is substituted for wheat bread and corn flakes are served for breakfast, if cereal is served." Sounds like a low-fat bonus, but if you have celiac disease, be careful of the corn flakes and be sure malt and malt derivations are understood as non–gluten-free when you book.

Virgin Atlantic (800) 862-8621

Forty-eight hours' notice will get you a gluten-free meal, but I have no idea what that is except the reassurance that "no wheat, rye, barley, or oats will be served and package labels will be provided if a food is served in a container. Starches include arrowroot, corn, potato, rice, or soybean products." This airline sounds as if it knows what it's talking about and it should, because celiac disease is a big deal in England. I would say taking pot luck with these people is a safe bet.

NOTE: Most airline personnel will heat up any special foods, i.e. corn muffins, bread or rolls, tortillas, etc., passengers on restrictive diets bring on board. The key is to ask nicely.

Airline Bottom Line:
Don't ask the airline what it has. Tell it what you want.

Sailing: The Finer Ports of Call

Did you know the word *posh* comes from the accommodations preferred by well-heeled British subjects crossing the Atlantic from Liverpool in the era of steamship travel? It stands for "port side out, starboard home," the side of the ship that afforded the savvy traveler relief from the blazing sun in each direction. It cost a pretty penny, or "bob," to be more precise, hence the term, which is now loosely defined as anything expensive and fairly snooty.

Ocean travel nowadays is no longer the floating exercise in class structure once favored by the Victorians, and it is no longer restricted to getting one, albeit the long way, from one place to another. Cruises can be wonderful, relaxing, invigorating, romantic, sophisticated, adventurous, educational, exciting, exotic, athletic, unforgettable, even slimming, and can take you absolutely nowhere and back, but whether you are traveling first cabin or on a deck lower down, no amount of money or connections will get you something to eat that's not on board when you set sail.

A week is a long time to be at sea without a cracker, and most cruises are longer than that. You can't exactly do a U-turn in the ocean and pick up a few things at the health food store, and a growling stomach doesn't do much for shipboard romance no matter how much moonlight dances on the water.

Good planning, on the other hand, can make for much smoother sailing. With plenty of notice, most cruise lines will accommodate any dietary need. Certainly not all the ships at sea will, but here are some notable examples.

AMERICAN HAWAII CRUISES (800) 765-7000

This cruise line says all special diets will be accommodated and suggests that prospective passengers send for or ask their travel agents for an American Hawaii travel book. It gives complete instructions and forms for requesting and securing all special diets, including wheat- or gluten-free with at least two weeks' notice.

CARNIVAL (800) 327-9501

Wheat- and gluten-free meals can be ordered through Carnival's medical department. All special requests must be made through your travel agent at least two weeks in advance. Representatives say it is a good idea to leave a note in the restaurant reminding everyone of your special requirements. I'd say that's a good idea on any boat.

COSTA (800) 462-6782

All special diets must be requested in writing to the Special Services Department at least two weeks before sailing. All necessary information will be faxed to the passenger or travel agent making the arrangements.

CRYSTAL CRUISES (800) 446-6620

This company will accommodate all special diets, including wheat- and gluten-free, but requests must be through a travel agent with a minimum of two weeks lead time. I'd give it more.

CUNARD (800) 5-CUNARD

The Cunard people run the Royal Viking and the Royal Viking Sun, where their chefs will prepare any special meals from galleys exclusively devoted to that purpose. A wheat- and gluten-free menu must be special-ordered at least one month before the ship returns to port and makes ready for the next sailing. It would be wise to make your requests directly to the ship company and through your travel agent.

NORWEGIAN CRUISE LINES (800) 327-7030

The people here draw the line at plum balls. No macrobiotic meals on this ship. But they will plan, prepare, and stock the foods for any other special diet, including vegetarian, kosher, low-fat, low-salt, low-sugar, and wheat- and gluten-free. With a minimum of two weeks' notice, they will even secure specific product brands, if necessary, and tell me they once had a passenger who could eat nothing but Oscar Mayer hot dogs. I'd start making them a list.

PREMIER (800) 327-7113

I am told the "Big Red Boat" has no way to handle special meals and recommends ordering via your waiter. The representative suggests eating a veggie diet while at sea, but I suggest calling the medical department at (407) 783–6061 before you blow them out of the water.

PRINCESS (800) 421-0522

"The Love Boat" loves a challenge. Special diets are listed on the passenger's record and gluten-free meals can be prepared with two weeks' or more notice prior to departure. It is recommended that you speak with the maître d' once on board to facilitate your request.

ROYAL CARIBBEAN (800) 327-6700

No special meal preparation is offered and no special diets of any kind are handled. The representative suggests asking your waiter to convey your requests to the kitchen on a meal-by-meal basis. I suggest there are other ports in a storm.

Other Possible Destinations

I've never been to a spa that didn't accommodate my gluten-free diet. If getting and staying healthy is not the point in these places, then where is it? As with everything, the trick is planning well in advance of your trip. If the spa is large, it is always a good idea to ask the manager to introduce you to the chef and explain your needs directly. After that, remember to ask the waiter to tell the chef where you are sitting and be prepared to wait an extra few minutes for your meal to find you. If you are very hungry and your food is taking awhile, which occasionally happens, remind yourself that waiting burns calories too and that you have gone to a spa to do just that.

Hospitals and psychiatric hospitals are trickier. You might not be conscious when your dinner arrives, or you might not notice it for any number of pharmaceutical reasons. It is always wise to have your doctor or a surrogate make your requests directly to the institution's nutritionist or dietician and alert the nursing staff that you could get a whole lot sicker if a cafeteria worker isn't paying attention and is too quick with the gravy ladle when your tray comes down the line. Anything can happen in a large institution where people routinely walk, roll, stagger, limp, crawl, collapse, and are carried in with the mistaken assumption that anyone in a white uniform automatically knows all their health problems.

One fact of hospital life you would do well to remember: If it's not on your chart, it doesn't exist. Have the nurse, doctor, hospital dietician, or nutritionist write "wheat-free diet" or "gluten-free diet" on your chart, preferably in red ink. It also doesn't hurt to carry something in your wallet that says you are allergic to wheat or gluten and that you require this medical diet under any circumstances. Obviously, if you are planning a baby or a nice, quiet nervous breakdown, you can tell the hospital about your diet yourself, but you never know when your gall bladder or the guy in the next lane is going to let go.

According to the Department of Defense, any person with a special dietary need that can be confirmed as a medical problem is disqualified from joining the army, navy, marine corps, air force, coast guard, national guard, or any other military service requiring a haircut and a uniform. It seems mess halls are not geared for special meals, especially during armed conflict. It would make no sense risking a person's life in battle, then killing him or her slowly with war rations. Anyway, who wants a medal for getting shot while hunting for rice cookies? In the event of a return of the draft or if there's a little flareup in New Jersey, your intolerance will be confirmed with a test.

If you are going to prison, your diet is probably the least of your problems. According to sources at my local state department of "big houses," it is important to contact the prison doctor. He or she will assign a special diet, which is then put in the computer and reviewed every thirty days—a routine, I am told, that is followed on the federal level as well. Other arrangements are made for "longer incarcerations," and officials would not comment when I asked what would happen to a grain-sensitive inmate caught carving a rice cake into the shape of a key. If you have to choose a last meal, wheat or gluten is the least of your worries.

In Case of an Emergency

You've done all you can. You've arranged your in-flight-on-board-on-track-on-deck special meal. You know how to say "I can't eat wheat or gluten" in several languages or, at least, you have packed the cards that will do it for you. You've read all the travel books. You've discovered the risotto regions of Italy, the best places in the Himalayas for lentil pancakes, and the rice belt on the Pacific Rim. What could happen? Anything.

Do not dial 911. American Express can't help. Turn to chapter 12 and look up the names and addresses of the support groups in the cities you are planning to visit. I hope they're all there when you need them. As of this printing, they were, but many of these people are volunteers, so it's possible for life to change, funding to dry up, what have you. If you do get an unanswered telephone, always ask the hotel manager to look up the group for you before you give up. The answer could be as simple as a change of address or telephone.

Do try. You never know. You might make a new friend or find the best loaf of brown rice bread in the world or that restaurant in the Marais in Paris rumored to be wheat- and gluten-free. Anyway, it's always nice to talk with someone who understands, especially when you are far from home and away from your own resources.

CHAPTER EIGHT

Etiquette for the Allergic

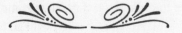

My method is to take the utmost trouble to find the right thing to say, and then to say it with the utmost levity.

— GEORGE BERNARD SHAW
from *Answers to Nine Questions*

Some years ago my husband and I had the good fortune to attend a dinner party for which the hostess had planned months in advance. We found ourselves at an impeccable table full of flowers, candles, gorgeous food, exquisite wine, and the perfect mix of people, the seating of whom had been considered with great care and with a certain mischief. The conversation virtually crackled with good cheer and interesting stories until someone at the other end of the gleaming, mile-long mahogany table, too far away for the subtlety of a whispered reply, asked my husband if it was true, as the man's dinner companion had pointed out, that he had recently undergone brain surgery.

It was, unfortunately, true. My husband had had surgery several months earlier to remove a tumor that would certainly have killed him if it had not been discovered. In fact, his jocular presence at that very dinner table was nothing short of a miracle. I had been hoping this festive evening would help both of us to begin to forget our recent trauma. I was not unaware of the frisson of tension that quickly took hold.

All conversation stopped. The guests waited. Soup spoons hung in midair. The hostess stared down at her plate and steeled herself for the pall that would surely settle over her lovely party along with the grisly details that would inevitably follow an affirmative answer. Sensing this and understanding that he held the success of our friend's evening in his power, my husband said nothing, merely smiled and appeared to be considering the path that would lead him out of the discomfort that had become palpable.

Finally, and with the infinite timing of a standup comic, he paused, gave the gathering his most wicked look, winked at our hostess who was growing paler by seconds, and said, "Brain surgery. Oh, yes indeed. I've just had one installed."

The room exhaled, the guests once again broke up into conversation groups, our relieved hostess smiled broadly, and we exchanged the look between husband and wife that says, "Well done."

Someone, it might have been Miss Manners, once said, "Etiquette is what you do for other people to make yourself feel better." Certainly knowing what to do in any given situation involves a great deal of empathy. No doubt, most social sins are committed not out of malice, ignorance, dimwittedness, thwarted toilet training, or any number of failings on the parts of our parents, but out of sheer self-centeredness and blind faith in the fact that everyone around us will be fascinated by the minutia of our suffering.

My husband saved that evening, not because he is the world's greatest wit, but because he knew that as soon as the question was asked, the evening needed saving. Rather than pointing out his fellow guest's rudeness at asking it in the first place and causing a different kind of discomfort, or muttering a long-suffering response meant to elicit pity for what was surely one of the most traumatic episodes of his life, he chose to save the man, his own privacy, and, most important, the spirit of *joie de vivre* our friend had worked so hard to achieve. He simply understood the situation from another point of view and gave the answer our hostess was praying for. He empathized.

It is said that Abraham Lincoln did this when the White House butler dropped the Thanksgiving turkey in full view of the guests.

With a conspiratorial wink at his guests and sparing the poor servant, he said, "Why don't we just serve the other one?"

George I was said to have abandoned his napkin and lifted his finger bowl to his lips when his guest, a chieftain from an African tribe, dined at court, showing all the snickering lords and ladies to be the snobs (did you know this word comes from the Latin *sans nobilite,* meaning "without nobility"?) they really were, proving the greater the man, the greater his courtesy. Good manners always include, never exclude.

A diet as restrictive as ours is not without its social cost, but I find the harder I work at helping others become comfortable with my problem, the more comfortable they, in turn, attempt to make me. The old saws were never truer: "To be loved, one must love; to receive, give; to have a friend, be a friend." I might add, "To be well hosted, host often and well."

So how do you prevent your presence at the dinner table from causing an allergic reaction all its own?

We are told manners today are meant to be flexible. Forget it. The following rules apply to any situation where you are not among members of your own family or very close friends who should know better.

Rule No. 1.

Always, always, always let your host know about your diet ahead of time.

This includes weddings, bar mitzvahs, showers, parties, suppers, lunches, barbecues, picnics—any meal prepared for you by someone else. There are no exceptions. Even if the person is a casual acquaintance and you are included in a large party, ask what is being served, either personally or through a closer friend. Always explain why you need to know and, if necessary, offer to supply your own food.

While it's perfectly acceptable to phone the bride and ask what is being served at a small reception at home, I'm not suggesting that you rush to the nearest phone if a large wedding is planned. Even if the bride is a brilliant neurosurgeon, she is most likely living on a cloud of tulle, arguing the fine points of the seating plan, ushers, flowers, music, or negotiating some other potential disaster that will make your call seem hopelessly selfish and badly timed. You have a choice here. Either eat first and nibble carefully at the reception or treat it like any large party.

When invited to any large party held in a restaurant, hotel, or catering establishment, phone the catering office and ask the person in charge of the event. These people know the dinner down to the last radish rose. You can't change the menu and it's extremely rude to try, but once you know what will be served, you will know whether you will need to eat before the party and how much or if slipping some extras into your purse or pocket would make sense.

At smaller parties that are catered in the home, it is perfectly acceptable to walk into the kitchen and ask the caterer what's in what's being served. The hostess probably doesn't know the answers to your questions, anyway, and is too busy being gracious to be bothered with them unless you seize up and topple into the pool. Who better than the cook to steer you in the right direction? In my experience, caterers love talking to guests, not only because they want to help, but because it's a great way to get more business. They certainly don't want you to get sick and mention their company's name.

A word of caution. Always be considerate of the caterer's responsibilities before asking your questions—the moment before twenty individual chocolate soufflés are to exit the oven and appear on the table is not an ideal one if you want a serious answer. It is not polite, nor is it attractive, to ruin everyone else's dessert just because you can't have one.

It's perfectly okay and, in fact, preferable to let your hosts know that you have done this. They will be relieved that you will not go hungry at their party, and you will be seen as supremely considerate, perhaps even worthy of another invitation.

Rule No. 2.

Never, under any circumstances, embarrass the host or hostess by announcing that you can't eat something he or she is serving.

If an offending substance finds its way onto your plate, say nothing. Simply slide it to one side, move it around, hide it in a pile of potatoes or behind other food or a utensil—under a nice big soup spoon is always good—or give it to the dog. Think about how creative you were disposing of Brussels sprouts as a kid and do the same thing, knowing you are not regarded with as much suspicion as you were then. Understand that no one but your dry cleaner will ever see the inside of your pockets.

If these and other diversionary tactics fail and you get caught anyway, try to be diplomatic. "It's my fault, I really didn't make myself clear. How could you have known, it took me years to figure out what gluten was. I'm perfectly fine, I had an enormous lunch." Then change the subject. "Speaking of pasta, how was your trip to Italy? . . . You know, these dumplings remind me of the twins. How are those darling chubby babies (grandchildren, godchildren, nieces, nephews) of yours?" You get the idea. If you don't, you won't be invited back. It's as simple as that. Hosts are not fond of guests who embarrass them.

When you phone the next day to thank the host (you always do that, don't you?) mention how sorry you are that you didn't explain your problem clearly enough. He or she may be too embarrassed to mention it, and you will be taking the heat off the host in the most gracious way possible. Unless the person is made of cement, you will be insuring it won't happen to you again because you will be providing an opening for the person to find out exactly what you can eat the next time.

It's never easy being a good guest, and it's even harder in your case.

Rule No. 3

Never, under penalty of death by pasta, answer the question "What happens when you have a little?" truthfully.

In this case, it is not a sin to tell a lie. If "You don't want to know" or "After making this beautiful (lunch, dinner, brunch, whatever), I don't think (name of host or hostess) would appreciate hearing about this just now" isn't enough to change the subject and stop any further questions cold, make it up.

Say when you have the tiniest bit of gluten, you are overcome with the urge to fondle warm rolls, bark, or break out in uncontrollable laughter, sarcasm, brilliance, a yeast infection, or "gluteny," so that you cannot control your compulsion to lick plates. Say you catch cold from the wheat germs or make up a story about cereal killing. Say anything but the truth and its gastrointestinal repercussions. No amount of coaxing or encouragement should delude you into thinking people really want to hear about this.

If the comment is funny enough, your inquisitor will soon forget the question, like you a whole lot better for the reply, and move on to another subject. This is not because the person has forgotten the question so easily, it's because most people really don't want to know the details, they just ask out of some odd social obligation to offer acknowledgment of the other person by expressing interest in what they really don't care about. Most people expect the other person to play by the rules and keep the answer as short and as interesting as possible.

If you're not sure this is true, remember the time someone asked you how you were feeling after that hernia operation and you told him in excruciating detail. You'll see that same frozen smile if you talk about your gastrointestinal tract at the table.

Of course, you never know. You may run into a gastroenterologist or a baker interested in developing a wheat- and gluten-free fudge brownie for the government person in charge of food labeling. In this case, make an appointment to discuss your problem somewhere less public. Of course, this rule holds true for social situations only. When a waiter asks you this question, the appropriate answer is "I'll get sick and die in this chair and my children will sue your children."

If you are invited time after time to a family table that does not acknowledge your special needs and you are convinced this is because they never liked you in the first place and now have a great vehicle through which to express that hostility, I say let your hair down and damn the consequences. That's what family therapists are for.

Rule No. 4.
Always eat a little something before going out to eat.

Scarlett O'Hara was told to do this. While antebellum society felt it wasn't seemly for a woman to be seen chowing down at a plantation picnic, your reason for doing the same thing should be obvious.

It's tough to be polite on an empty stomach. In fact, there's a strong potential for rudeness when you arrive at a party and find there's nothing for you to eat. Your ability to hold up your end of the conversation and your responsibility as an interesting and lively guest really take a nose dive when your stomach is growling.

Even if you think you know what is being served, an evening out can hold some nasty surprises for people whose food is restricted, and spending an evening in a constant state of starvation is a rough way to learn. I once went to a traditional Italian Christmas Eve "Frito Misto" party thinking this was food I could eat and discovered absolutely everything was battered and fried.

There were many guests, and good manners dictated that I keep my mouth shut and the items on my plate moving. My dinner consisted of cheese, nuts, and so many cups of espresso, I was up until New Year's. When I got home, I ate everything in my refrigerator, including the baking soda and the spare batteries.

Think of it this way: If you've eaten already and there is nothing for you, you'll survive without being tempted to cheat or punch a newly papered wall. If you've already eaten and there's plenty for you, your willpower and self-control in the face of calories and fat will become the envy of all present and the buzz of the next day's postparty gossip. Talk of your self-possession and strength of character will precede you wherever you go. With a reputation for restraint to uphold, it won't be difficult to lose those last five pounds either.

No matter how you look at it, if your stomach is full, you can't lose. If it's empty, you can't win.

Rule No. 5.
Never forget to say thank you.

This should go without saying. Alas, it's amazing how few people say thank you anymore.

Whether it's a chef who has prepared your special pasta, a pal who has remembered your rice crackers for the cocktail party, the weekend hostess who combed the health food store and found your special bread so you could have your breakfast toast and jam, or, the ultimate demonstration of love, the person who made you a loaf of bread from scratch, never accept these gifts—and make no mistake, they are gifts—without conveying your gratitude.

I don't mean the immediate reflex of saying thank you, which of course will be sincere and heartfelt at the time. I'm talking about a follow-up note, fax, phone call, card, flowers, or even a gift, depending on your budget and the extent of your gratitude. I always send a note of thanks to a chef who has gone out of his way for me. (Phone calls are not always appreciated in chaotic restaurant kitchens.) I do this not merely because it is the gracious thing to do, but because in these times of moving fast and forgetting one's manners, it virtually insures that I will enjoy more of that special treatment.

Here, too, there are no exceptions. Your note doesn't have to be formal, expensive, stylish, or even particularly well written, just sincere. My personal favorite is a postcard, usually a funny photograph from the forties or fifties involving food, such as classic diners and drive-in burger stands, old TV shows such as *I Love Lucy, Father Knows Best,* and *Donna Reed,* and vintage advertising postcards. I collect them by the dozens.

When someone makes or buys something special for me, I simply flip through my stash and send the one that most fits the occasion. After a while, matching the postcard to the kindness becomes a game, and it has become my trademark thank you. You'd be surprised at how much food you can find on a postcard.

Browse through the tables of old postcards and photographs at the flea markets. Look for food advertising and pictures of appliances, toaster assembly lines, cake mixes, refrigerators, ovens, muffin tins, and the like. There is no need for formality. If you have as much fun saying thank you as you had enjoying the result of someone else's effort, it is impossible to go wrong.

It doesn't matter what you send or how you send it, as long as you never forget to do it. When you follow up with some tangible expression of your gratitude, you salute the generosity of your friends and express your own graciousness, refreshing behavior in these less than gentle times.

You also may be surprised that something as small as a note or a postcard can open the door to a new friendship. Some years ago a stranger brought me a gift of corn pasta when our visits to the home of our mutual friend coincided. It was absolutely unnecessary and all the more appreciated because it was, which is exactly what my note said. If you make a habit of meeting every act of generosity, no matter how small, with the generosity of your own appreciation, you will soon realize the more you say thank you, the more reasons you will have for doing so.

A person who says thank you is always welcome. Simple as that.

Rule No. 6.

It is impolite to mistake a business breakfast, lunch, or dinner for a meal.

Business has its own etiquette or, perhaps more accurate, its own *non*etiquette. To be brash and rude and ignorant of the basic pleasantries is to be considered dynamic, powerful, plugged in. Witness Barry Diller, Lawrence Tisch, Donald Trump.

It is an unspoken rule that no one ever eats at a power meal or, if so, eats as little as possible. I think this is to create the impression that to be truly powerful, one must be beyond the need for food, but willing and able to expense it.

Conversely, the need to eat seems to conjure images of weakness and corporate wishy-washyness. Eating heavily at business meals can arouse the predator in the meekest accountant, and I would advise against it. I don't know why, but the amount of food left on one's plate seems to correlate directly to one's position in the hierarchy—the more, the higher.

This can work to the benefit of the grain intolerant who must do business over a meal. Eat a hearty breakfast at home—rice cereal, tapioca toast, jam, and gluten-free pancakes—narrow your eyes, square your shoulders, order a fruit salad or a small glass of orange juice, and drink lots of coffee or tea. It's also good to be perceived as impervious to caffeine. Ditto for lunch and dinner straight from the office. Have a peanut butter and rice bread sandwich at your desk and nibble a salad or take two bites of an omelet with the boss or the client.

Whatever you do, don't discuss your problems with wheat or gluten over drinks. One minute you're bonding, the next you're being passed over for that beer account or the new pretzel business. Speaking of which, no one ever has to know you're not drinking because of the grain. Drinking during business hours these days is tantamount to corporate suicide. Fizzy water is the way to go here.

For larger office gatherings and morale-boosting events such as picnics on the boss's lawn or taking over an entire bowling alley, eat first and wing it. When no one is looking, trade plates with your spouse, or if this is an employee-only party, transfer small amounts of food (just enough to avoid arousing suspicion) into the plate of the person on your left. Keep doing this until yours is empty.

I'm not suggesting everyone with whom you work is a cutthroat out for your job, and certainly some lifetime friendships have been known to bloom among colleagues and clients, but in the shrinking ranks of today's business world, it's wise to be known for something other than your intolerance to certain foods.

When I worked for a large advertising agency fond of working lunches in the conference room, I explained my problem to the office steward. I asked that whenever he saw my name on a luncheon meeting list, he serve me something from the list I provided and suggested he keep in the galley.

Another way to eat well without having to talk about it is to put in a standing lunch order at a nearby restaurant and ask that it be served to you when you come in with colleagues or clients. The added benefit here, of course, is being asked, "The usual, ma'am?" Big points with the power types for that.

Another simple strategy is to make a study of take-out places near the office that offer enough for you to eat. Keep a list of them in your desk and pass them out to anyone who might be asked to arrange for your food to be brought in.

Bottom line: Be as gracious to business colleagues who serve you special foods as you are to friends and try to make sure you have enough to eat at all times. The idea is never to make a big deal of it. If you're like most people in business today, you've got quite a bit on your plate, none of which has much to do with food.

Rule No. 7.
In your case, it is polite to carry your own food where other food is served or sold.

This means restaurants, diners, snack bars, athletic stadiums, beach houses, cabins, cottages, mansions, apartments, lofts, church suppers, picnics, barbecues, lunches, brunches, boats, Greyhound buses, airplanes, trains, trolleys, trailers, parlor cars, vans, sedans, station wagons, recreational vehicles, national parks, country clubs, swimming pools, sidewalk cafés, bistros, malls, movie theaters . . .

. . . anywhere eating is allowed in the first place and as long as you do it with discretion and flair. That is, it is *not* polite to crack an egg on the back of a movie seat, but it is perfectly acceptable to slip a cookie or some wheat- or gluten-free candy out of a purse or pocket.

It is perfectly acceptable to hand your bread to a waiter and ask that it be returned in the form of French toast, eggs Benedict, or a Reuben sandwich or a double cheeseburger, but it is *not* acceptable to do so without benefit of a plate. It's tacky to clutter the table with plastic bags and napkins full of crumbs.

It is absolutely acceptable to transfer the contents of a ready-made sandwich to your bread in a public place, as long as you don't make a mess or call unnecessary attention to what you're doing.

When you have been invited to someone's home for the weekend, by all means, arrive with a suitcase full of your special food. But don't expect to be waited on hand and foot. Just because you have a problem with grain doesn't mean you can't operate a toaster or a microwave or open a box of cereal.

Whenever you carry your own food, it's important to let those in charge know what you're doing ahead of time. Movie managers sometimes have rules about bringing food into their theaters where popcorn and other snacks are sold. Of course, you are an exception, but if you don't want a scene with an usher and to risk being treated like a sneak eater, which actually happened to me, mention that you will be doing this and why. With competition from videos as fierce as it is, what movie house in its right mind is going to rule against you?

While it is perfectly acceptable to eat your corn muffin instead of the one served by the restaurant, remember it is rude to eat it before everyone else is served. No matter how hungry you are, you are not exempt from basic table manners. Comments such as "Boy, am I glad I have this gluten-free roll" when everyone else is starving are rude, mean, and totally rotten.

Rule No. 8.
It is acceptable to use your fingers when all else fails.

"All else fails" is the operative phrase here. If you are served a cracker on which there is a single, small piece of cheese or meat, it's fine to pick it up with your fingers and pop it into your mouth. If that cracker is loaded with something gooey that you can eat, find yourself a plate, fill it up, and eat the parts you can with a fork or spoon.

Never attempt to deconstruct a canapé with your fingers.

If you were smart enough to bring your own crackers, now is the time to fill up a plate and make the switch somewhere other than the buffet table in the center of the room. Afterward, do not leave the uneaten ones lying around on a windowsill, next to someone's purse, or behind a photograph of the family dogs. Someone will find them eventually and know it was you. The more often this happens, the less likely your name will appear on a subsequent guest list. Ask a catering employee to dispose of them or do it yourself as neatly and as quickly as you can.

If you've come to this party with your own spoon, heap small amounts of each item onto a cocktail plate, and enjoy the food from there. Never, under any circumstances, put your spoon directly into the serving dish. Always use a utensil from the table to serve yourself, and use your spoon only to eat your portion. If there is no powder room to rinse your spoon discreetly, ask the bartender for a glass of water and use that, remembering not to leave that glass around either.

If you find yourself at a sit-down dinner, staring down a chicken that has been fried or otherwise coated with something that is not wheat- or gluten-free, remove the skin with a knife and fork, leave it in as small a pile as you can manage, then lift the leg or the breast or the wing to your mouth with your fingers.

Should an offending grain find its way into your mouth, there is always your napkin. Pray it's paper. Use it to dispose of the food, then dispose of your napkin immediately. Attract as little attention to yourself in the process as you possibly can. I like to pretend I've dropped something, then quickly duck under the table to insure privacy.

If you can time this maneuver to avoid bursting out laughing, you're doing well.

In summary: Your diet doesn't excuse you from applying all the basic rules of courtesy and social conduct and, in fact, requires that you learn some new ones. When in doubt, smile. If you are really in doubt, buy yourself a copy of Emily Post or Miss Manners. And never do anything in polite company involving food, wheat-free, gluten-free, or otherwise, that you would not like to read about in the morning paper.

CHAPTER NINE

Your Cheating Heart and Other Special Problems

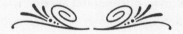

You always hurt the one you love.

—THE MILLS BROTHERS

You will want to cheat. And you will.

This is not a four-week-ten-pounds-off diet. This is for life, and therein lies the problem.

In the beginning, there is denial, which is not a river in Africa. You will stash cookies in kitchen drawers. You will have a Big Mac attack and eat the roll. People will wonder why the front seat of your car is full of crumbs, why your briefcase smells of prune Danish and pepperoni pizza, why there are chocolate chips in your bed. In the middle of the night, you will shave the sides of a lemon pound cake as I have, telling yourself the thinner the slice, the safer the serving.

You will feel the urge to cheat most strongly when you are flying through time zones. Airborne and among strangers, I imagine my problems are suspended and I am in a kind of free zone where gluten has no effect on me. I am always saved, though, by comparing the pallid roll or petrified muffin on my tray to the Viennese pastry or the crusty baguette waiting for me on the ground. I postpone the peril for something worth getting sick over. I must confess, I have had two self-inflicted relapses since my own diagnosis of celiac sprue, one that can be traced to a vacation in Cape Cod and gallons of corn and lobster bisque and another home alone with a truffle cake sent for Christmas by a well-meaning, but unenlightened, business associate. I may be weak and disgustingly human, but I am proud to say, even in desperation, I have my standards.

You will hate the people who try to stop you, even if those people are those nearest and dearest. It's normal for people who love you not to want to see you become ill again and to become quite upset when they witness what they know is a deliberate attempt to do yourself in with a bagel. This, in turn, will upset you because, as everyone knows, a good defense is a good offense, and anyone who has ever watched the daytime talk shows also knows it is impossible to save another person from self-destruction and it is foolish and unenlightened to even try.

If you cheat enough, some of your more sophisticated friends might even try an intervention, which is really a confrontation during which everyone who loves you will take turns telling you how sad they are that you are eating wheat and gluten. No matter how people choose to let you know you are doing something dangerous, you will meet their anger with your own, you will insult them and accuse them of trying to control you, and a fight will ensue. Everyone will remember the whole episode as dumb and stupid, but then so is cheating.

Even when your family and friends think your actions stem from ignorance, absentmindedness, or a temporary lapse in judgment, they will automatically assume you want to be saved, which, as you know in your cheating heart, is not always the case.

The world can be a dangerous place for people like us, and it is very hard to resist the temptation to cheat that comes with travel, especially to countries where eating your customary foods brings with it another kind of peril.

Anticheating Strategy No. 1
No matter how much you might regret it later, tell your traveling companions and tour companions about your diet.

Tell them before the urge to cheat hits, in the airport while you're waiting to board the plane. (You did order a gluten-free airline meal, didn't you?) Carry nibbles for your room or on the road, pack something sweet of your own for dessert. Offer them any bread or sweets that come with your meals. If you are traveling alone, break all the rules of etiquette and tell total strangers more than they want to know about your diet—the flight attendant, the person sitting next to you, the waiter at your hotel, the manager of room service. Who cares what they think? You'll never see them again.

When it comes to vacations, the danger is not restricted to staying in hotels, getting to and from a place, or even attempting to order new and odd-looking foods in foreign countries. Any vacation from a routine and the responsibilities of work for more than a long weekend qualifies as a potential trouble spot, even if that means sitting on your own front porch with a pile of books or sleeping in your backyard hammock for an entire week.

Vacations are extremely tricky. We work hard, save our money, fly to Disney World, book a cruise, or rent a cottage in the woods. We drive, fly, hike, bike, sail, or swim off and forget all our worries and restrictions for a few weeks. We overspend, overeat, overplay, overindulge ourselves, our kids, our spouses, our friends; even the dog comes home with a T-shirt he'll never wear. We overdo it all, vainly trying to squeeze out two weeks of pleasure among fifty weeks of pain.

Restraint doesn't seem to have much of a say on vacation because the word *no* never seems to make it into the suitcase. I think this is because holidays are so hard to come by and are so tied up with feelings of deserving.

How often have you overheard one vacationer say to another about an ice cream sundae, a Mai Tai, or a Rolex, "Oh, go ahead, you deserve it . . ."? How often have you said this yourself? My point exactly. Trouble is, what you deserve is not necessarily what is good for you.

Anticheating Strategy No. 2
Pack your own wheat- and gluten-free cookies, cakes, pies, and pizza, eat too much of them, and come home as fat and guilty as everyone else.

Life's Big Moments are also fraught with every emotional opportunity to cheat. Phrases such as "Hey, it's my birthday," "It isn't every day you get married . . . turn fifty . . . retire, celebrate fifty years in the armed forces, get divorced, have a baby, join a convent, get arrested, win the lottery, land a part in a movie" are dead giveaways that there is trouble ahead.

To make matters worse, it is virtually impossible to attend or be the guest of honor at any of these occasions without prolonged exposure to cake, especially if you happen to be the bride or the groom and have let your in-laws talk you into a wedding cake you can't eat. I don't even want to think of the lifetime of concessions in store for the person who can't or won't make demands on his or her wedding day. (If this is the case, reread chapter 3 immediately!)

Anticheating Strategy No. 3

See how many noncake festive desserts you can invent. (Anniversary rice pudding, the "I-Can't-Believe-I'm-Fifty" hot fudge sundae, bon voyage flan, individual baby shower meringues, retirement bombe, rehearsal dinner torte, and the divine wedding dacquoise just to get you started.)

This may sound odd, but funerals are dicey for cheating potential. I think it's because food is so central to the process of grieving. Mountains of food and enough leftovers help ease the burden for the family by getting them through the first difficult days.

How do you explain your wheat and gluten problem to a person who has just lost a loved one? You don't. You put something on your plate for appearances and before you know it . . . it's gone.

Anticheating Strategy No. 4

Don't bother the bereaved or similarly preoccupied person with your problems. Just bring a nice wheat- and gluten-free covered dish, keep your hands out of the bagel chips, and say something nice about the deceased. This strategy works for floods, hurricanes, tornadoes, earthquakes, nuclear explosions, acts of war, and other natural disasters as well.

Job pressure is another big obstacle to self-control, especially the insidious variety found at the average about-to-be-downsized corporation. Everyone is paranoid about everyone else. The boss says "Jump" and a chorus answers, "How high?" The boss says "Let's go for burgers" and before you know it, you're tucking into a double cheese-burger on a sesame seed bun. You tell yourself you're doing it in the name of bonding and job security.

Tell yourself this: No one has ever been fired for refusing to eat bread. If you are, you probably have a landmark case.

Anticheating Strategy No. 5
Tell the boss about your wheat or gluten intolerance and just happen to mention how important strict adherence to your regimen could be in the containment of health insurance costs to the company.

Working late with nothing but a vending machine, a few take-out menus, and a hole as big as Cleveland in your stomach also can be devastating, but easier to handle. Keep a box of your cereal, crackers, rice cakes, and something that packs a big protein wallop, such as peanut butter, in your desk for the next time. Make sure you wash your utensils carefully, wipe jars, reseal packages, and close lids tightly; it won't be good for your career to be seen spraying Raid into your drawers or listing "desk extermination" among your business expenses.

If you're lucky enough to have a private office big enough for more than the basics, I would strongly advise buying a small refrigerator and keeping it stocked. Otherwise, using the one in the employee lounge or cafeteria will do, as long as you label your food with as much guilt-producing poignancy as possible. "Please don't steal this. It's the only food I can eat!" is always effective.

Anticheating Strategy No. 6
Figure out how many hours are lost to the company while your coworkers are out having pizza. Contrast this to the cost of a refrigerator, a set of safety seal storage containers, and a bread crisper for your office.

Cocktail parties and big buffets are always dangerous. In your case, a moment on the lips is not a lifetime on the hips but a lifetime of annoying intestinal snips. If the idea of repeating this experience isn't enough to deter you, arrive so full you couldn't manage to pop a shrimp puff if you tried.

Sometimes even the tiniest twinge of deprivation can push us over the line and trigger a cheating episode—anger, happiness, sadness, boredom, thirst, water retention, success, failure, gloom, loneliness, envy, apathy, feelings of abandonment, loss of anything from a loved one to one's keys, being loved too little, too much, or not at all, even the discovery of a few unwanted pounds, a particularly nasty bout of PMS, a fight with the boss, or a full-blown midlife crisis can weaken our resolve and leave us facedown in a plate of chocolate chip cookies.

It's impossible to control something you don't understand, so it's important to discover what motivates the urge to cheat. Is it real hunger, which usually announces itself suddenly, loudly, and often painfully? Or is it emotional hunger, which creeps up on you and doesn't seem to have much to do with the need to fill your stomach at all?

Physical Hunger

Physical hunger is not a rational thing, but rather an irrational, animal one that lives in the dark and tangled pit of our stomachs and speaks to us in the low, rolling growl of need. True hunger does not respond well to dos and don'ts, shoulds and should nots, or diet restrictions of any kind, especially one that bans the glutinous belly fillers that satisfy it so quickly. Like Popeye, the hungry stomach "wants what I wants, when I wants it."

If you are truly hungry, the sight of any food, including those off-limits on a wheat- and gluten-free diet, will trigger an uncontrollable urge to consume. Sadly, there are many people in the United States who experience this kind of hunger every day. And every day, the rest of us get up and go to our refrigerators because we only think we do.

Anticheating Strategy No. 7
Understand that the way to your cheating heart is through your stomach. Keep it reasonably full at all times, not so bursting full that you get fat and acquire other problems, but just full enough to keep your brain from sounding the eating alarm.

Emotional Hunger

There is an old saying in diet circles: "It's not what you're eating, it's what's eating you." Unlike physical hunger, emotional hunger is not so easy to appease. The stomach rarely growls. There is no sudden pang, no sharp pain propelling you into the kitchen. Something else, far more primal, moves us to this kind of eating. If in addition to simple appetite appeal, the food we are considering carries with it feelings of love, warmth, happiness, fullness, satisfaction, comfort, and safety, if it stirs memories of any kind and it also contains wheat or gluten, it may be virtually impossible to resist.

Emotional hunger is insidious. It creeps up on you while you are watching television, in the middle of an argument, during a moment of sadness and loss, when you have too much work and too little time, when you have the flu, a broken foot, tennis elbow, poison ivy, or whenever you feel most sorry for yourself. It arrives with your divorce papers, the new car agreement, the mortgage application, the promotion, or the pink slip. It can explode in a sudden desire to eat everything in sight, and it can show up right after a filling meal because emotional hunger doesn't come from the stomach, but from the heart or the head or the psyche. It comes from wherever we keep our pain.

Like anything that comes from deep within your emotional programming, this kind of hunger is a powerful force. One minute you are a normal person eating three wheat- and gluten-free meals plus snacks a day, and the next you are chowing down an entire pizza with everything on it or working your way through a box of glazed doughnuts, an emotional hostage, hating yourself more with every bite.

If you don't spend some time figuring out which emotions or situations cause this kind of irrational response in you, you will always be imprisoned by it, destined to cheat on your diet without knowing why.

Unexamined emotional hunger often is the reason people become obese, alcoholic, drug addicted, fools in love, abused, and worse. It's why you have no idea why you would even consider doing serious harm to yourself with a spring roll. Yours is no different from more obvious forms of self-destruction, it's just that wheat- and gluten-free diet abuse isn't juicy enough or sick enough to make it to the talk shows. Regardless, you must take your problem just as seriously.

Compounding this and under the surface of what appears to be our national and public preoccupation with healthy eating, moderate exercise, and normal body weight is a blitz of media messages that bombard us with images that do not add up and speak in subliminal ways to the stay-hungry, never-too-thin, size-two-and-obsessed images some of us still harbor in our private and hungry hearts. Every day we turn on our televisions and see too many people eating far too much to be so thin.

Anticheating Strategy No. 8
Forget "you are what you eat." Remember "you eat what you feel."

There are as many behavioral cues in one's life as there are breaths in each day, and it would be impossible to discuss the derivation of every impulse, but the following chart may help you see the big ones and apply the lessons to your own personal list of emotional land mines. When a truck hits you, it's very important to get the license plate and a good description of the driver. It's just as critical to know what's driving your behavior and to understand the difference between what's felt and what's real. While these interpretations may not always apply to you, they should offer some serious food for thought.

Feeling	Reality
My life is empty.	My stomach is empty.
I can't have anything.	I can't have this corn muffin.
I want to crunch a pretzel.	I want to bite your head off.
I'm so angry, I could eat everything in the house.	I have trouble expressing my anger, so I eat bread instead.
I need pasta.	I need a hug.
I want to hurt you.	I am hurting me.
Others try to control me.	I see assistance as control.
I need to eat this pie.	I need attention.
You don't care if I eat this cookie.	I need to talk about why I want to eat this cookie.
If I get sick and die, then you'll love me.	If I get sick and die, no one will love me.
Why me?	Why not?

On closer introspection, you may find that the various feelings behind the urge to cheat express themselves in the need for different foods. If you watch and listen carefully, you may be able to match the food craving with the feeling. It's different for everyone, but these may strike a familiar chord.

Pretzels, chips, bread sticks	=	Anger
Pasta, noodles	=	Sadness
Cocktail mix nibbles	=	Denial
Ice cream, anything frozen	=	Pain
Muffins, toast, cereal	=	Romantic love
Gravy, stuffing, sandwiches	=	Mother love
Anything Entenmann's	=	Unrequited love
Bite-sized cookies, nuts, M&M's, large amounts of miniature food	=	Anxiety

I know a rather unusual therapist who holds the revolutionary view that the only trouble with most people is that they've never learned how to suffer. He says we have dedicated our entire culture to the notion that psychic pain is preventable and have erected a culture of denial around the misguided belief that if we try harder, we can deflect or postpone or even wipe out this necessary human condition.

Building on that hypothesis, one could say that most self-destructive behavior is a subconscious unwillingness to acknowledge what is really going on; that it is a repetitive and futile attempt to avoid the unfamiliar territory of our own feelings and to be enlightened by lessons our experiences can teach us.

If you doubt this, all you have to do is watch someone dating the exact same person he or she just divorced to see what great and destructive lengths people will take to avoid learning something about themselves through their angst. Still unconvinced, watch an angry ex-smoker light up after a fender bender in the parking lot.

A friend of mine is fond of saying about life "No one gets out of it alive." Isn't it easier to stop spending enormous amounts of energy on the struggle to remain unaffected by our suffering and just give up, feel the pain, and get on with it, maybe even learn something in the process?

Anticheating Strategy No. 9
Suffer.

The next time you experience sadness or hopelessness or anger and you feel like crying, slamming a wall, whining, or hollering your fool head off, find a private place and do it.

Let your feelings happen, instead of keeping them under a tight lid. If you're unaccustomed to doing this, you will become extremely uncomfortable during the first few minutes of this exercise. Resist the impulse to push your feelings away. The whole process shouldn't take more than fifteen minutes. My guess is that when you find out what's really going on, you will no longer want a bagel.

Anticheating Strategy No. 10
Make a stack of photocopies of the following "cheat sheet" and fill it in every day for two weeks.

Patterns will emerge. Associations will be made. A particular time of day may reveal itself to be more dangerous than another, one activity more fraught with more temptation than another. The results may surprise you.

In this journal do whatever it takes to tell the truth. If you ate standing up, say so. The more specific you are, the more insight you will gain, the more control over those times you are most susceptible to going off your diet.

Whenever you begin to lose touch with the emotions that drive your cheating behavior, make some fresh copies and start over, and don't fall into the oldest trap of all. Always begin by forgiving yourself for the indiscretion that may have prompted your fresh resolve and avoid the downward spiral of one episode of cheating leading to another, then another.

Anticheating Strategy No. 11
Acknowledge your cheating with forgiveness. And start fresh.

You know how this goes: "I've already had half a pie, so why not be a total idiot and finish it off?" This, of course, is followed by: "I feel

DAILY CHEAT SHEET Date _____

	Foods Eaten	Time Eaten	Where Eaten	With Whom	In response to physical hunger? (Rate level from 1 to 10)	In response to emotional hunger? (Rate level from 1 to 10)	Symptoms
Breakfast							
Midmorning Snack							
Lunch							
Afternoon Snack							
Dinner							
Miscellaneous food consumed (List of all picking, nibbling, noshing, vendor food. Remember, eating over the sink, cleaning plates, and finishing the kids' sandwiches count!)							

_____ I did not cheat at all today.
_____ I cheated a little today.
_____ Wheat and gluten disaster

_____ I resolve to forgive myself the weaknesses of today and to start again tomorrow, committed to my health, determined to end my self-destructive behavior and to be as resourceful in finding wheat- and gluten-free foods I will enjoy as I am in finding the foods I sneak.

_____ Not perfect, but better than before. I will try harder tomorrow.

_____ Congratulations! Keep up the great wheat- and gluten-free work.

Comments:

sick now because I'm bad, so why don't I eat something really bad and make it worthwhile getting sick over?" Blah. Blah. Blah. Blah. It doesn't matter whether you're talking about pounds, as in "I'm already fat; why not get fatter?" or offending substances: "I'm already miserable; why not be really miserable?" It all comes down to being able to stop the cycle by acknowledging your very human failings and forgiving yourself. Viewed this way, weakness itself can become a strength.

Dieting: The Double Whammy

Many people are malnourished when they are diagnosed with celiac sprue or wheat allergy. Once diagnosed, the emphasis is on rebuilding health, strength, and muscle, which means resuming a normal body weight, which in turns means eating pretty much anything you want for a while.

At five feet eight inches and a whopping ninety pounds, hair cropped to about an inch all around to encourage new and healthier growth, my husband dubbed me "Q-Tip with Chocolate Shake."

The trouble is we eventually *do* gain weight.

Some people do this gradually over a long period of time, slowing down at what is easily maintained, but others just keep on gaining. The experts say this is due to a combination of calories, grams of fat, level of activity, age, and whether the metabolism is still racing or it has been turned down by the thermostat of time. Weight gain can even depend on how badly or how well the body absorbs, based on how little or how much damage the intestine has sustained during the active phase of the grain intolerance.

I have my own theory on the subject, of course, and it's simple. What is unattainable is suddenly attractive. People who rarely ate bread, cookies, pasta, or pie now can't get enough of the wheat- and gluten-free varieties. We are loading up on foods we never ate in the first place, just because we can't have their mainstream counterparts.

Like many young women in the 1960s and 1970s, I associated carbohydrates with unwaiflike, unfashionable figures. I nibbled cottage cheese, fasted occasionally, ate hard-boiled eggs or bananas, and black coffee day after day and attributed my wafer-thinness to good genes and exceptional willpower. Now I never miss a meal and rarely pass up the opportunity to enjoy a new gluten-free muffin or cookie or pasta dish, and, like everyone else in America over the age of consent, I find I must diet.

Dieting is never easy, but for people who know eating just enough gluten to develop symptoms is the quickest route to skin and bones, it can be a tempting reason to cheat, kind of like having your cake and eating it too. Don't be shocked. I know you've thought of it.

Anticheating Strategy No. 12

Find a really terrible photograph of yourself taken while you were sick. The next time you are tempted to eat pasta in order to lose weight, make note of your rib cage pushing through your shirt, your sunken eyes, your lackluster skin. Remember how sitting at your desk bruised the "buttons" on your back. Understand that there is such a thing as being too thin.

While today's diets are a far cry from the ketosis-producing high-protein diets such as Stillman and Scarsdale and others that all but guaranteed a rebound the minute normal eating was resumed, the new emphasis on long-term changes in eating habits, limiting consumption of red meat, increasing one's fiber and decreasing dependency on fat, and losing a more conservative pound or two a week is undeniably healthy. However, the new low-fat diets can be dangerously low on fat, a substance we need small amounts of in order to maintain a good working body. They also rely heavily on complex carbohydrates. While this may be easy and even a pleasure for most people, it can be very dangerous for people like us.

Liquid diets are not only unrealistic—the minute you eat real food, you regain the weight—they are particularly dangerous for people with wheat and gluten problems. If you can find one of these potions in a flavor that contains no wheat or gluten, you are doomed to consume only that flavor, reducing an already impossible diet down to its barest bones. This cannot be good for you.

The organized weight-loss programs are no better. You can't eat the convenient frozen dinners made by Weight Watchers and sold in supermarkets, even though you can follow the diet offered at local centers.

Forget Jenny Craig or Nutri/System or any of the self-contained programs available only at franchised centers. Food labeling laws do not apply to products that are sold privately. Not only will it be difficult for you to find something you can eat, you will have no idea how many calories and grams of fat each meal contains for when you're ready to go it alone.

Many of these companies count on your regaining the weight. When your bottom line expands, so does theirs. Enough said?

The Dean Ornish program (the whole deal; not the book) is considered so heart healthy, it is the first weight-loss program to be considered reimbursable by a major health insurance company—Aetna. While this is good news for normal folks and I can say I have enjoyed watching friends literally melt away before my eyes, their middle-age hearts throbbing with new vitality, I have serious concerns about this plan for wheat- and gluten-intolerant people. This vegetarian diet is heavily grain-dependent, and I don't think it makes good nutritional sense to eliminate a second food group by choice when another is off-limits by medical decree. With so few grains available to us, there is a huge opportunity to cheat on this diet. Frankly, I don't think it's worth the risk.

If you have recovered so well that you now have a weight problem, my advice is to lay off the gluten-free desserts for a while, count calories, cut down on portions, watch the fat, and start a moderate exercise program. Before you embark on any program, see your family doctor or your gastroenterologist. In fact, I would strongly advise newly diagnosed people not to go it alone when starting a wheat- and gluten-free diet, but to seek professional nutritional counseling in the person of a registered dietician and seriously plan your diet with an eye to complete recovery. (This means inside as well as outside.) Dropping in from time to time for a professional update can't hurt either.

The same goes for those of you who need to put some more meat on your bones. Forget those high-calorie shakes and power powders. They're full of chemicals and hidden grains as well. Eat more well-balanced meals and keep taking those vitamin supplements, especially B_{12}.

For those of you who insist on following the latest fad, I am happy to report that those new thigh creams are wheat- and gluten-free.

Thank You for Not Smoking, Drinking, or Eating Red Meat, Fats, Sugar, Caffeine, and Chocolate

Any form of self-imposed deprivation, act of willpower, or abrupt change in lifelong patterns can put a severe strain on your carefully maintained equilibrium and trigger a wheat or gluten cheating episode. It really doesn't matter what you give up or why—cigarettes, alcohol, artery-clogging fats, diet sodas, animal protein, or lollipops. One big no-no in your life is enough. Two can put you over the top. During the first two weeks of any voluntary deprivation, it is very common to experience the urge to shift addictions. Experts report that recovering drug addicts begin drinking, reformed drinkers suddenly crave chocolate bars, eschewers of fat yearn for sugar, and so it goes. Here's how to make sure you don't move from cigarette puffs to puff pastry.

Anticheating Strategy No. 13
Get rid of every no-no in the house. Serve only wheat- and gluten-free meals. Send the family out for breakfast, lunch, and dinner, if necessary. It's only a couple of weeks. How hard could it be for them?

Anticheating Strategy No. 14
Never try to tough it out alone.

Tell everyone around you what you are giving up and why, and ask for their support and understanding before you start. Join a support group or start an informal one of your own. Find a like-minded friend and do it on the buddy system. Confess that you might want to cheat on your wheat- or gluten-free diet and ask to be saved ahead of time.

Anticheating Strategy No. 15

Take up needlepoint. Or weaving. Or painting. Or juggling.
It is impossible to eat cookies while doing these things.

This may sound silly, but you can't eat bagels if your hands are busy with something you really enjoy. I don't count months and years when I speak of my own success at staying off cigarettes, nor do I tell horror stories of eating English muffins while caught in the throes of withdrawal. I count pillows and chair covers and beach bags and eyeglass cases.

Whether you have told yourself there is no flour in a certain dish you simply had to have, just nibbled the edges of a cookie, or walked into an Italian restaurant in broad daylight and brazenly ordered a heaping bowl of linguine and clam sauce, there is one final thought that may help.

Anticheating Strategy No. 16

Remember that success is only getting up one more time than you fall down.

You're only cheating yourself.

CHAPTER TEN

Twelve Chefs Take the Challenge

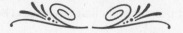

Give me the luxuries of life and I will gladly do without the necessities.

—FRANK LLOYD WRIGHT

With apologies to George Herbert on the subject of what is the best revenge, living well cannot hold a cannelloni to eating well. The discovery of a densely rich chocolate torte made in the classic way with no flour but rather with finely ground almonds is enough to send people like us straight to heaven. A light and creamy ricotta cheesecake on a pedestal of ground, gluten-free cocoa cookies can reduce us to tears. All that I own, I gladly give for gluten-free lasagne laden with cheeses and fresh tomato sauce.

Thanksgiving, the most carbohydrate-intensive of all the family feasts, no longer has to be the turkey of holidays it is for people like us when there is pumpkin pie enrobed in a crust of gluten-free ginger cookies, one of the tastier reasons to be thankful, nor does it have to be a constant round of "no thanks" when you make the apple and sausage stuffing or your own family favorite with cubed and toasted brown rice bread, your own bread mix, or crumbled corn bread you have baked yourself.

Christmas used to be the clanging Ghost of Puddings Past until I realized that if I cooked the meal, I controlled the meal, and no one would ever again say to me "Oh, you can't eat that, can you?" You can bite the heads off all the gingerbread people you want when you bake them yourself with any one of the fabulous mixes out there. No more picking the sponge cake out of the trifle either, or giving the pfefferneuse, the sugar angels, and the chocolate Santa cookies to the dog.

Once you get over feeling deprived and find out how well you really can eat in spite of your wheat or gluten restriction, you may even find you have added a dimension you hadn't bargained for, one that could even require a quick detour to a health spa or gym to shed the extra pounds such unchecked bliss will surely encourage. (Not to worry, most spas will cater to your wheat- and gluten-free diet.)

The evening I prepared Angelo Peloni's creamy and classic risotto swimming in butter and Parmesan cheese was the day I could face the fact that I would never eat semolina pasta again. The night I discovered that my Philadelphia neighborhood restaurant, the wildly popular Judy's, would gladly use my own gluten-free pizza crust to make their grilled veggie, mushroom, and sun-dried tomato pizza with goat cheese that rivaled any I remembered, there was fresh proof of how far a little creativity and some determination can go.

And when I gave Sheila Lukins a box of Pastariso with a request for "real spaghetti and pasta sauce, the kind I miss most," I understood how far a big hunger and a willing chef can take the concept of culinary happiness.

I have yet to run out of ideas for toppings for the thick pizza crust Bette Hagman taught me how to bake. I keep an extra in the freezer at all times, right next to the gingerbread muffins, Beth Hillson's truffle brownies, and the store-bought gluten-free waffles I have discovered can be the foundation of everything from a simple breakfast to a wonderful dessert laden with fresh strawberries and towers of whipped cream.

I, for one, am tired of perky-sounding recipes meant to placate the poor soul who can't have the real thing, doomed by their cuteness, fooling no one. I don't enjoy endless conversations about whether vanilla extract is poison or quinoa is in or out of favor, nor do I enjoy eating my food from a plastic bag while everybody else eats theirs from a plate. This is boring, self-defeating, depressing, and dumb, and it's not my idea of dinner. Give me something fabulous, something everyone at the table will love, *then* tell me it's wheat- and gluten-free.

That was the challenge given to the talented chefs who appear in this chapter. The recipes that follow prove that not only can this be done, it can be done brilliantly and with the same genius showered on food lovers everywhere. The recipes are far from fat-free, they do not contain calorie counts or the fat, protein, and carbohydrate contents per portion, and there has been no attempt at nutritional balance. The fact is, you don't want to know how many calories lie on the next several pages. I advise you to invite friends to share the bounty or suffer the consequences.

These foods are for the soul, not the waistline. They are meant to inspire and to encourage you to ask your own neighborhood chefs to share their secrets, adapt their recipes, and maybe even create some new ones just for you. There are plenty of cookbooks to help you stay slim, heart healthy, holistically correct as well as wheat- and gluten-free. Virtue is not the point here. I will leave that to the angels and your conscience.

These are the foods you miss most, desserts you only dream about, comfort foods you thought you had to forgo forever—a gorgeous corn and lobster pie in a chili-polenta crust, a variation on the lasagne you've been longing for, two divine pasta sauces, a decidedly grown-up baked macaroni that appeals to your inner child's need for comfort, the queen mother of all chocolate tortes, biscotti, risotto, a sweet corn soufflé straight out of Georgia O'Keeffe country, a delicate fruit tart that tastes like clouds, a richly satisfying Italian dumpling called gnocchi, and a Thai-jita that blends the fire of the Orient with the flavors of Mexico.

I'd be hard-pressed to find better culinary minds to put to the task of creating great wheat- and gluten-free dining than the impressive group gathered here, but I'd also find it difficult to find a more generous group. These twelve inspired chefs, food writers, entrepreneurs, and restaurateurs not only represent the best cooking talent in America today, they represent the nurturing spirit of giving that moves people into the kitchen in the first place.

To paraphrase that awful French woman, "Let 'em eat biscotti . . . and torte and tarts and Thai-jitas and gnocchi and spaghetti and soufflés and macaroni and risotto and lasagne!"

Herewith, twelve chefs take the challenge.

Sheila Lukins

There aren't many kitchens in America that do not have at least one, and most likely all three, of the books Sheila Lukins coauthored as founder/chef of the Silver Palate. Anyone who doesn't remember the phenomenon of red and white jars and bottles of the same name multiplying on every department, specialty, and gourmet store shelf in the decades that followed surely must have been out of the country for quite a while. Today, as food editor of *Parade* magazine, the talented and peripatetic Ms. Lukins has just produced the glorious *All Around the World Cookbook* (Workman, 1994) and is about to publish another.

It's a miracle she had time to cook for us at all. With the great generosity of spirit that is her trademark, she has produced a pair of beautiful pasta sauces, one a tribute to bold summer flavors, the other smooth and winter hearty, both a complement to the slightly nutty flavor of Pastariso brown rice pasta (if this is not available in your health food or gourmet market, see chapter 12) or your own wheat- and gluten-free favorite.

Cold Sauce "Hot Stuff" Pasta

Summer is the season of easy meals, unexpected guests, and vivid vegetables bursting with flavor. Meant to be served cold, this zesty sauce takes advantage of all three and is easily made ahead. All you need do is boil up the pasta according to package directions and toss before serving.

Serves 6.

- 2 red or yellow bell peppers
- 6 cups tender fresh spinach or arugula, washed, tough stems removed
- 1 cup pitted imported black olives, coarsely chopped
- 1 large clove garlic, finely minced
- 1 tablespoon finely grated orange zest
  Fresh black pepper to taste
- 1 2-ounce can anchovies, drained
- ⅓ cup extra-virgin olive oil
- 8 ounces fusilli or rice twists
  Coarsely grated fresh Parmesan cheese (optional)

1. Halve, core, and seed peppers. Flatten lightly with palm of your hand. Line a baking sheet with foil.

2. Lay peppers skin side up in a single layer on baking sheet. Place under a preheated broiler, 3 inches from heat source. Broil until skins are charred black. Remove to a plastic bag; seal it well for about 15 minutes to steam. Remove from bag and slip off and discard skins. Cut peppers in ¼-inch strips lengthwise.

3. Place the greens and olives in a large bowl. Sprinkle with garlic, orange zest, and black pepper.

4. Cut the anchovies in half and add to the greens. Toss the mixture with the olive oil.

5. Before serving, cook the pasta al dente in a pot of boiling salted water. Drain; rinse under water. Toss with the spinach mixture. Sprinkle with cheese, if desired. Serve immediately.

Pasta Rustica

This winter sauce is hearty, smooth, and studded with tomatoes, bell peppers, raisins, capers, and olives. Serve it on a chilly night with a simple winter green salad and a crusty loaf of homemade rice bread. It will delight and warm everyone who shares it.

Serves 6 to 8.

   5 tablespoons extra-virgin olive oil

1½ cups thinly slivered yellow onions

   2 red bell peppers, cored, seeded, and cut into ¼-inch strips

   2 tablespoons coarsely chopped garlic

   2 28-ounce cans Italian plum tomatoes

   2 tablespoons tomato paste

   1 2-ounce can anchovies packed in oil

   1 cup pitted green olives, halved

 ½ cup golden raisins

 ¼ cup drained capers

   2 teaspoons dried oregano

 ½ teaspoon hot red pepper flakes

     Salt and coarsely ground black pepper to taste

 ¼ cup plus 2 tablespoons chopped fresh flat-leaf parsley

   1 pound dried "spaghetti-style" rice pasta

1. Heat 4 tablespoons olive oil in a heavy saucepan over low heat. Add the onions and cook for 10 minutes until wilted, stirring once or twice.

2. Add the bell peppers and garlic. Cook, stirring, over low heat another 10 minutes.

3. Coarsely chop the plum tomatoes with their liquid and add to the vegetables along with the tomato paste. Cook, stirring once, for 5 minutes.

4. Coarsely mash the anchovies and add to the pot with their oil. Mix in the olives, raisins, capers, oregano, pepper flakes, and salt and pepper. Stir the ingredients together and simmer over medium-low heat for 30 minutes, stirring occasionally, until piping hot. Add ¼ cup parsley and cook for 1 minute longer.

5. While the sauce is simmering, bring a large pot of water to a boil with a pinch of salt and the remaining tablespoon of olive oil. Add the pasta and cook until al dente. Drain the pasta and divide between 6 to 8 pasta bowls. Top with the sauce, and sprinkle on the remaining 2 tablespoons of parsley. Serve immediately.

NOTE: This sauce is also delicious over roasted fish or chicken.

Molly O'Neill

No matter that I moved away from Manhattan more than fifteen years ago, my Sundays still belong to the *New York Times*. The slow, ritual reading of the paper, the hoarding of my favorite sections for last, beats most offers of mimosas and eggs Whatever hands down. As a celiac I have no desire to witness the relentless gobbling of croissants and the buttering of muffins that are a part of weekend brunches.

I'd rather read, clip, circle, mark for more serious follow-up, make note of who died and of what, and who got married on the St. Regis roof, remark on the silly clothes being worn on the street, and muse aloud on the rise and fall of the dollar and the crime rate, lazing my way through the *Book Review* and the *Magazine* until that final sweet moment reserved for Molly O'Neill's Sunday rhapsody on food.

The following recipe is not one of those meal-on-the-table-in-an-hour deals. It is not inexpensive. It requires the husking of fresh corn, the steaming of lobsters, and the coddling of a custard in something the French call a *bain Marie*, a method of resting one pot in another filled with water and cooking in the oven. It also requires the freshness of summer ingredients and, if at all possible, a sunny kitchen with a porch overlooking an endless and blue ocean, waves of Puccini floating in the background.

If not, the act of creating such a beautiful dinner as this can transport the cook, as it has me, to this perfect summer place in the heart. With gratitude to my favorite paper, reprinted by permission, copyright 1994 by The New York Times Company:

Corn and Lobster Pie in a Chili-Polenta Crust
from "Play It by Ear" by Molly O'Neill

Serves 6.

POLENTA

2¾ cups water
⅔ cup yellow cornmeal
1 teaspoon chili powder
¾ teaspoon salt
Freshly ground pepper to taste
Olive oil spray (nonalcohol)

CUSTARD

3 large cloves garlic, unpeeled
2 eggs
1 cup milk
1 teaspoon salt
Freshly ground pepper to taste
Kernels from 2 large ears of corn

LOBSTER MIX

Kernels from 1 large ear of corn

2 lobsters, steamed, tail and claw meat removed and cut into ½-inch dice

1 red and 1 yellow bell pepper, stemmed, cored, deribbed, and cut into ¼-inch dice

1 jalapeño pepper, seeded and minced

1 tablespoon chopped fresh cilantro

2 scallions, chopped

1 tablespoon fresh lime juice

½ teaspoon salt, plus more to taste

Freshly ground pepper to taste

1. *To make polenta:* Bring water to the boil in a medium saucepan. Stir together the cornmeal, chili powder, and salt and pepper. Whisking constantly, add the cornmeal mixture to the water in a slow, steady stream. Switch to a wooden spoon, lower the heat slightly, and cook, stirring constantly, until the mixture is very thick, about 25 minutes. Spray a 9-inch pie plate with the olive oil spray and spoon the polenta into it. Place a large sheet of plastic wrap over the polenta and press it out with your hands to cover the bottom and the sides of the pie plate evenly. Remove the plastic and set the dish aside.

2. *To make custard:* Preheat oven to 350°F. Wrap the garlic in aluminum foil and roast until soft, about 45 minutes. Lower the temperature to 325°F. Peel the garlic, place it in a mixing bowl, and whisk to puree it. Add the eggs and whisk lightly. Add the milk and salt and pepper, and whisk just until well combined. Stir in the corn. Pour the mixture into the polenta shell. Place the pie plate in a large roasting pan and fill the pan with enough hot water to come halfway up the sides of the pie plate. Bake until the custard is set, about 1 hour.

3. *To make lobster mix:* Toss together the corn, lobster, bell peppers, jalapeño, cilantro, and scallions. Add the lime juice, salt, and pepper. Taste and adjust the seasoning, if needed. Spoon the mixture evenly over the custard. Cut the pie into wedges and serve immediately.

Alex Cormier

If you blink, you'll miss Alex Cormier's tiny restaurant. Alex on South is tucked away on Church Street in the bucolic New Jersey town of Lambertville on the Delaware River just across the bridge from the tourist bustle of New Hope, Pennsylvania.

The first time I lunched in his restaurant's vest pocket garden, I steeled myself for the moment I would be forced to cast my eyes away from a tray of exquisite desserts that would inevitably make its way to my table. When the waiter began to tell the story of the financier, an almond-flour torte topped with caramelized fruit and baked in a ring resembling a wedding band, which he said was originally served at engagement parties during the reign of one Louis or another, I realized there was no need. Alex himself traces the roots back to New York and Le Cirque Restaurant. We may never know its true origin, but I do know this, the financier looks more complicated than it is.

Banana Financier

You will need eight four-inch financier rings (use them later for tarts or your mail-order English muffin mix), which are available in restaurant supply stores, good kitchenware shops, or Jamesway stores, and a cookie sheet large enough to accommodate them comfortably. If the rings are not available, cookie cutters, approximately four inches in diameter and two inches high, will work just as well.

If almond flour is not available, finely ground pistachio or hazelnuts will do nicely. It is also possible to double the batter, which will keep, refrigerated, for a week. I freeze the unadorned financiers for finishing another day. Serve them on very special occasions with your own spin on the tale.

Makes 8 individual tarts.

BATTER

- 8 eggs
- ½ pound (2 sticks) unsalted sweet butter
- 1 tablespoon gluten-free vanilla extract
- 2⅔ cups almond flour, ground as finely as possible. (See note.)
- 1 cup sugar

BANANA TOPPING

½ cup sugar

4 bananas, sliced in half lengthwise and in half again crosswise

1 tablespoon butter

1 bar of the silkiest, most sinfully rich chocolate you can afford, slivered, shaved, or broken into small chunks
Powdered sugar, whipped cream, crème fraîche, or sour cream

1. *To make the batter:* Separate the egg whites and reserve the yolks for another purpose. Melt the butter in a skillet over medium heat until it's light brown, taking care not to let it burn. Remove the skillet from the heat as soon as you see the butter turning brown. Let it sit. This will give the batter its nutty flavor.

2. Mix the almond flour, sugar, and vanilla in a bowl. Add the egg whites to the mixture and whisk with a spoon or whip to combine the ingredients. (Mixing ten to fifteen times should do it.) Add the brown butter and stir.

3. Leave the batter in the refrigerator overnight or for at least four hours.

4. *To make the topping:* Place the sugar in a skillet over medium heat. Stir constantly with a wooden spoon until it caramelizes and turns a lovely light brown. (The entire process will take between 30 and 40 seconds, so this is not the time to answer the phone.) Once the sugar is browned, add the bananas and cook another 10 seconds on each side. Add 1 tablespoon butter and remove from the heat immediately. (The butter will stop the cooking process.) Toss to coat the bananas evenly and let the mixture cool to room temperature.

5. *To assemble:* Line a cookie sheet with parchment, baking, or waxed paper and arrange the financier rings on the sheet. Spoon batter into each ring approximately three-quarters full. Spoon the banana mixture over the batter to fill each ring. Divide the chocolate equally and sprinkle over each ring.

6. Bake at 450°F. until firm and lightly browned, approximately 12 to 15 minutes. Watch carefully. Use a sharp knife or cake tester to make sure the financier is firm in the middle. Before letting it cool,

remove each tart from the ring by carefully running a sharp knife around the sides. Remove from the cookie sheet and remove tarts from the rings by running a knife around the sides again. Let cool on rack.

7. Just before serving, dust with powdered sugar or, if you prefer, top with a dollop of whipped cream, crème fraîche, or sour cream.

Variations

If you are willing to experiment, this tart can be the basis for many desserts. Try it with whatever fruits are in season or on hand. Fresh peaches, kiwis, raspberries, blueberries, blackberries, papaya, and mango are particularly good, and the combination of pear slices and chocolate can only be described as heaven on a spoon. Chef Cormier does not recommend strawberries, however, because their water content can result in a soggy financier.

NOTE: To make almond flour, toast ½ pound whole unblanched almonds on a baking sheet at 400°F. until brown. Grind them in a coffee grinder or in a spice mill. (A food processor will give you almond butter!)

Ed Barranco and George Georgiou

Chef's Market opened its doors on Philadelphia's South Street in 1983, and, ever since, partners Ed and George along with their executive chef, Kevin Smith, have been raising the level of eating, shopping, grazing, foraging, indulging, knoshing, nibbling, and sidewalk sitting well beyond the standard set by its less freewheeling neighbors to the north. The food is dished up with a healthy serving of local gossip, goodies for the tourists, and a willingness to accommodate yours truly's need for glorious gluten-free food at any time of the day or night.

With their compliments, here is the Chef's Market version of Mexican Lasagne adapted from *The Frog Commissary Cookbook.* It really fits the bill when you crave the taste of something spicy and yearn for the rich texture of something gooey and Italian. My family calls this "the Pearl Harbor of Lasagnes." One minute, you're pleasantly full, going back for seconds, then wham, the zeroes scream in and you're sunk. Alert your tailor. This dish is rich.

Mexican Lasagne

This recipe is time-consuming, with prep time about thirty to forty-five minutes and cooking time another forty-five, but everything but the final assembly can be prepared in advance, including the crème fraîche. The dish freezes well and the results are well worth every ounce of effort required.

Save this one for the weekend when you're not rushed. As long as you're going to the trouble, you'll thank yourself for dividing the uneaten portion into individual servings for a quick meltdown in the microwave on one of those days when removing your shoes sounds like too much work.

The recipe provides eight hefty servings accompanied by nothing more complicated than a salad of mixed greens.

Serves 8.

CHICKEN LAYER

1½ cups of chicken stock
 2 teaspoons crushed coriander seeds
 6 bay leaves
 1 pound boneless, skinless chicken breasts cut into
   1-inch strips
 ¼ teaspoon salt
 ½ teaspoon pepper

BEEF LAYER

 ¾ pound ground beef
1½ teaspoons ground coriander
 ⅛ teaspoon ground cloves
 ¼ teaspoon pepper
 ½ teaspoon dried oregano
 ½ teaspoon ground cumin
 1 teaspoon minced garlic
 ¾ teaspoon salt
 2 tablespoons minced roasted jalapeño peppers *or*
   ¼ teaspoon crushed red pepper flakes
 2 tablespoons gluten-free vinegar

ONION MIXTURE

2 tablespoons olive oil
3 cups thinly sliced onions
½ teaspoon salt
2 4-ounce cans mild green chilies, chopped

TOMATO SAUCE

4 pounds ripe tomatoes
2 tablespoons olive oil
1 tablespoon minced garlic
2 tablespoons sugar
1¾ teaspoons salt
½ teaspoon pepper

ASSEMBLY

18 5-inch tostados (corn tortillas fried until crisp in
   ½-inch corn oil, then drained well)
3 cups crème fraîche *or* 3 cups sour cream mixed with
   3 tablespoons lemon juice and 2 beaten eggs
1 pound Cheddar cheese
1 tablespoon minced fresh coriander *or* parsley
   A handful of pitted and sliced black olives

1. *To make chicken layer:* Combine the stock, coriander seeds, and bay leaves in a deep skillet and bring to a boil. Simmer 5 minutes. Add the chicken, cover, and again bring to a boil. Reduce the heat to very low and cook 7 to 10 minutes more, or until the chicken is just done.

2. Pour the contents of the skillet into a sieve set over a bowl to catch the broth. Let the chicken cool. Return the broth to the pan and reduce the liquid over medium heat to ½ cup. Set aside. Remove any bay leaves and seeds from the chicken and cut the meat into ½-inch pieces. Combine the chicken with the reduced broth and the salt and pepper. Set aside.

3. *To make the beef layer:* Combine all the ingredients in a skillet. Cook over medium heat until the beef loses its pink color and the vinegar has evaporated. Set aside.

4. *To make the onion mixture:* Heat the olive oil in a 9-inch skillet.

Add the onions, salt, and chilies. Cook over medium heat for about 10 minutes, stirring frequently. Set aside.

5. *To make the tomato sauce:* Preheat the oven to 475°F. Put the tomatoes stem side down in a single layer on a rimmed baking sheet lined with aluminum foil. Bake for 25 to 30 minutes, or until the skins are lightly charred.

6. Puree the tomatoes, skins, stems, and all, and then put them through a sieve. Heat the olive oil in the skillet. Add the garlic and sauté for about 15 seconds. Add the pureed tomatoes, sugar, salt, and pepper. Cook, stirring occasionally, over medium heat for 10 to 15 minutes, until the mixture has thickened. Set aside.

7. *To assemble the lasagne:* Preheat the oven to 350°F. Lightly oil a 9 × 13 × 2-inch baking dish. Put down a layer of 6 tostados. Mix the chicken with half the onion mixture and 1 cup tomato sauce. Spread the mixture over the tostados. Drizzle on 1 cup of crème fraîche or sour cream. Sprinkle 1 cup of the cheese. Lay down 6 more tostados, pressing and flattening down the layer below. Combine the beef with the remaining onions and 1 cup tomato sauce. Spread this over the tostados. Top with 1 cup crème fraîche or sour cream mixture and 1 cup Cheddar cheese. Lay down the last 6 tostados and the remaining cheese.

8. Set the pan on a rimmed baking sheet and bake for 35 to 45 minutes, until golden and bubbly. Let the lasagne rest 15 minutes before serving. Garnish with sliced black olives, coriander, or parsley.

Beth Hillson

Beth Hillson's response to her own diagnosis of celiac disease was to rush off to culinary school and add "fabulous chef" to her list of credentials as food and travel writer. Since then she has produced two more milestones in the history of grain intolerance—one is a newly diagnosed six-year-old named Jeremy, who has to be the luckiest celiac alive, and the other is a very successful mail-order business called the Gluten-Free Pantry, where she creates some of the best baking mixes imaginable—sinfully good concoctions such as Chocolate Truffle Brownies, Country French Bread, and Orange Walnut Biscotti, among others. Some say her white bread mix is the closest you can get to the yeasty, chewy real thing, and her bagels were the toast of a recent *Good Morning, America* show. This is a woman who truly believes in eating as the best revenge. And she proves it tastefully.

When Beth isn't mailing brownies or pancakes to grateful people or tucking wheat- and gluten-free treats into Jeremy's backpack, she is exploring new territory—experimenting.

Pumpkin Prosciutto Gnocchi

"Gnocchi?" say most chefs. "It'll never happen without wheat flour to hold it together." Beth Hillson doesn't take no for an answer. The textural secret to this northern Italian cross between pasta and a dumpling is in just the right mix of rice flour, potato starch, and xanthan gum.

Brava, Beth!

Serves 4 to 6.

1 cup minus 2 tablespoons white rice flour
4 tablespoons potato starch
1 teaspoon grated fresh nutmeg
½ teaspoon xanthan gum
½ teaspoon salt
Freshly ground pepper
Pinch sugar
1½ cups pumpkin puree (canned or fresh)
¼ pound (1 stick) melted unsalted butter
⅔ cup ricotta cheese (check labels)
4 tablespoons Parmesan cheese
2 eggs separated
½ cup finely chopped prosciutto
Extra Parmesan cheese

1. Combine the rice flour, potato starch, nutmeg, xanthan gum, salt, pepper, and sugar. In a medium mixing bowl, combine the pumpkin puree, 4 tablespoons of the butter, ricotta and Parmesan cheeses, and egg yolks. Fold in flour mixture. Fold in the prosciutto. In another

small bowl, beat the egg whites until they form soft peaks. Gently fold the whites into pumpkin mixture. Chill 30 to 60 minutes.

2. Bring 6 to 8 quarts of water and 1 tablespoon of salt to a simmer. Shape spoonfuls of the chilled mixture into 1-inch balls. Gently drop the balls into the simmering water. Cook, uncovered, for 5 minutes, or until the balls puff slightly and feel somewhat firm to the touch. Using a slotted spoon, lift the gnocchi out of the simmering water and set on a paper towel–lined platter to drain.

3. Pour 2 tablespoons melted butter into a shallow serving dish and swirl to coat it with the butter. Gently transfer the gnocchi to the dish in one layer. Drizzle with remaining 2 tablespoons butter and sprinkle with Parmesan cheese. Serve immediately.

John Rivera Sedlar

John Sedlar grew up in Santa Fe, but his heart as well as his deeply creative spirit is rooted just north of there in the pueblo of Abiquiu. There his grandparents Eloisa and Pablita settled, ran the family ranch, and introduced him to the wild herbs, piñons, pumpkins, squash, apricots, corn, chili, beans, tortillas, and biscochitos that became his culinary inspiration. They have resulted in an interpretation of Southwest cuisine that can only be described as stunning.

Author of *Modern Southwest Cuisine* (reissued by Ten Speed Press, 1994), esteemed member of *Food and Wine* magazine's Honor Roll, and the driving force behind the newly "haute" tamale, this master chef/ artist leaves out no detail that fails to delight the eye as well as the palate, designing the gorgeous oversized plates that serve as backdrop for his astonishing food himself. From the Abiquiu restaurant in San Francisco and the newest Abiquiu in Santa Monica, which has just opened to rave reviews, and with credit to James Foran, here is his magnificent corn soufflé, which elevates the modest kernel to art and proves that spectacular desserts are only as far away as a chef's imagination.

Abiquiu Hot Corn Soufflé

If you are so inspired, serve this dessert as Chef Sedlar does, with passion fruit and caramel corn. If not, a dollop of pureed raspberries and a drizzle of chocolate sauce will more than do nicely.

Serves 6.

Butter and sugar for preparing the baking dish
8 ears fresh corn
¼ cup milk
⅛ cup sugar (or ¼ cup for more sweetness)
1 egg yolk
⅛ cup rice flour
1½ cups egg whites (12 eggs)
¼ cup sugar

1. Preheat the oven to 400°F. Generously butter and sugar a 2-quart ovenproof ramekin or soufflé dish and set aside.

2. With a knife, remove the kernels from the ears of corn. Put the kernels in a blender and pass through a fine sieve. Measure 2 cups of corn puree into a medium saucepan and stir in the milk. Place over medium heat and bring to a simmer.

3. In a medium bowl, whisk together ⅛ cup of the sugar (or ¼ cup for a sweeter soufflé) and the egg yolk, then add the rice flour and whisk again. Continue whisking while pouring the heated corn mixture over the yolk mixture.

4. Return the mixture to the saucepan and place over medium heat. Bring to a boil, stirring constantly until ready to use, about 15 minutes.

5. Just before final assembly, whisk the egg whites with ¼ cup of the sugar until soft peaks form. Gently fold the egg white mixture into the cooked corn mixture and pour into the buttered and sugared ramekin. Level the mixture off the top of dish and clean the sides. Place the dish in a larger pan and fill the larger pan with water until it reaches halfway up the side of the ramekin.

6. Bake, watching carefully, for about 13 minutes. When the soufflé has risen, serve immediately.

Jim Burns

Jim Burns, coauthor of *Women Chefs: Portraits and Recipes from California's Culinary Pioneers* (Aris/Addison Wesley, 1987), editorial director of *The Best of New York* from the Gault Millau Guidebook Series (Prentice-Hall, 1990), winner of the Lowell Thomas Award for excellence in travel journalism, now editor of the FoodStyles Feature Service of the Los Angeles Times Syndicate, is allergic to wheat. It can cause him everything from general flulike fogginess to an all-out debilitating malaise, depending on how much or how little finds its way onto his plate.

Jim is also committed to exploring the brave new world of alternative flours, experimenting with new combinations of ingredients and techniques, discovering new recipes, and featuring them in his column for other less talented, but equally tormented, souls.

Thai-jitas

Unlike traditional Mexican fajitas, which are based on tortillas, these Thai-jitas require rice wrappers, which Asian grocery stores carry in two sizes. You'll want the smaller version, which is about six inches across. While you're there, pick up the clear variety of nam pla (fish sauce), not the creamy one. Nam pla is very salty, so don't add salt to this dish. Be warned. The fire in this recipe comes from Thai chili paste. If you're used to milder foods, adjust down from 1 tablespoon to 1 teaspoon of paste. If you don't own a wok, don't rush out and buy one. Any large, deep-sided sauté pan will do.

Makes 9 Thai-jitas.

- 1 pound shark, tuna, swordfish, or other firm fish
- 1 tablespoon canola oil
- 1 teaspoon sesame oil
- 1 onion, sliced
- 1 sweet red pepper, cored and sliced
- 1 sweet yellow pepper, cored and sliced
- 2 tablespoons nam pla (clear fish sauce)
- 1 tablespoon Hoisin sauce (See note.)
- 1 tablespoon Thai chili paste
- 1 package rice papers
- 9 fresh cilantro sprigs

1. Wash the fish in cold water. Pat it dry and cut it into 1½-inch strips.

2. Heat the canola oil in a wok over high heat until almost smoking. Add the fish strips and cook until just done, about 5 minutes. Set the fish strips aside and drain all liquid from the wok.

3. Add the sesame oil to the wok and heat. Add the onion and cook 2 minutes. Add the peppers and cook another 2 minutes.

4. Mix the fish sauce, Hoisin sauce, and chili paste in a small bowl. Stir the mixture into the vegetables, and continue cooking. Add the fish and mix well. Remove the wok from the heat.

5. Take 1 rice paper at a time and dip into a bowl of warm water until pliable, about 10 seconds. Shake the excess water back into the bowl. Set the rice paper on a plate and place about 3 tablespoons of the fish-vegetable mixture down the center. Add a cilantro sprig and roll into a cylinder. Repeat the process.

Eggplant Variation
Makes 12 Thai-jitas.

    2 tablespoons nam pla (clear fish sauce)
    1 medium eggplant, unpeeled and cubed
    1 tablespoon Hoisin sauce (See note.)

1. Place the fish sauce and eggplant in a saucepan and set over medium heat. Cook, stirring occasionally, until the eggplant reaches a pastelike consistency, about 10 minutes. Stir in the Hoisin sauce. Remove the pan from the heat.

2. For each Thai-jita, fill each rice wrapper with ¾ eggplant filling and ¼ fish/pepper filling.

NOTE: Jim can tolerate Hoisin sauce, but for those who cannot tolerate even a trace of wheat or those with celiac disease, leave it out. It's nice but not necessary to the enjoyment of this dish.

Nick Malgieri

This man knows his way around dessert. He also knows the one true way to a grain intolerant's heart is through the pastry cart. Author of *Nick Malgieri's Perfect Pastry* (Macmillan, 1989) and *Great Italian Desserts* (Little, Brown, 1990), he has literally written *the* book for lesser mortals as well as for aspiring professionals—he is the creator of the baking section of the New York Restaurant School's textbook. When Signore Malgieri is not traveling, lecturing, directing the baking program at Peter Kump's New York Cooking School, writing recipes for *Chocolatier*, *Cuisine*, and the *New York Times*, he is editor of *Pasticceria*, a publication of the Italian Trade Commission, and the American correspondent for the Italian magazine *La Pasticceria Internazionale*.

Does this master baker ever sleep? Not until the biscotti are perfect.

All-Corn Biscotti

These are a wheat- and gluten-free version of the delicate and crunchy biscotti napoletani. The chef suggests you let the dough cool after the first baking or it will be difficult to cut into the individual biscotti. I suggest using a sharp knife, oiling your hands very lightly to press sticky dough into the pan, and sealing the biscotti in an airtight container to keep them crisp.

Mille grazie, maestro!

Makes about 6 or 7 dozen biscotti.

- 2 cups whole, unblanched almonds
- 1 cup yellow cornmeal
- 1 cup cornstarch
- ½ teaspoon baking soda
- ½ teaspoon cinnamon
- 1 egg
- ⅔ cup sugar
- ¼ cup honey
- 2 tablespoons melted butter or vegetable oil
- 1 teaspoon gluten-free vanilla extract

1. Preheat the oven to 350°F. and set a rack in the middle level. Butter a 13 × 9 × 2-inch pan and line the bottom with parchment or foil.

2. Place 1 cup almonds in a food processor fitted with a metal blade. Grind finely by pulsing repeatedly. Place the ground almonds in a medium bowl with the remaining whole almonds, cornmeal, cornstarch, baking soda, and cinnamon. Stir well to mix.

3. In a separate large bowl, whisk the egg. Whisk in the sugar, honey, butter or oil, and gluten-free vanilla. Add the dry ingredients and stir with a rubber spatula to form a stiff dough.

4. Scrape the dough into the prepared pan and press with the palm of your hand to form an even layer about ½ inch thick, completely covering the bottom of the pan.

5. Bake for about 30 minutes, until well risen and firm. Cool in the pan for 5 minutes, then invert to a cutting board and cool completely.

6. Cut into three 3 × 13-inch strips, then cut each strip into ½-inch slices. Arrange biscotti on cookie sheets or jelly roll pans and bake again for about 15 minutes.

Caroline Winge-Bogar

Carrie will soon pack her stockpots, saucepans, casseroles, wooden spoons, wire whisks, spatulas, gratin dishes, and her newly minted degree from the Culinary Institute of America and head for the Norman Rockwell town of Carlyle, Pennsylvania, where she will trade the old Cup O' Joe café sign for a new one that says Atlas World Cuisine.

Along with her *batterie de cuisine* and a feel for the foods of a simpler, more innocent time will be her husband, Jerry, and a two-year-old named Scout, who could be the reason Carrie is probably the only chef in America who is not afraid to show what she can do with Rice Krispie treats and macaroni and cheese. "It's a better place to raise a family, build a life, find great 1940s and 1950s furniture, spend the Fourth of July," says the young mother of her new home, as I imagine an entire town opening its top button, letting out its collective waistband.

Grown-up Macaroni and Cheese

No Leave It to Beaver *supper, Carrie's version of macaroni and cheese is what a memory tastes like on a very sophisticated tongue. A decidedly grown-up combination of Brie, Muenster, and provolone provides the melting proof this dish can hold its own at any dinner party.*

Forget fat grams. This supreme cheesyness is something you miss more than Bosco. The Bogars are slim. Theirs is the metabolism of youth combined with the frantic schedule of a restaurant and that of a small boy. They'll have their turn.

Serves 4.

- 1 10-ounce box of Pastariso elbows
- 2 tablespoons cornstarch
- 1½ cups milk
- 1½ cups half-and-half
- ¼ pound (1 stick) butter
- 4 ounces Brie, cut into a medium dice
- 2 ounces Muenster, cut into medium dice
- 2 ounces provolone, cut into medium dice
- 2 egg yolks
- ½ teaspoon salt
- ½ teaspoon coarsely ground black pepper
- 2 slices of "bread," chopped in food processor, *or* packaged wheat- and gluten-free crumbs (optional)

1. Preheat the oven to 350°F. Prepare the elbows according to package directions to al dente, taking care not to overcook.

2. Combine the cornstarch with 2 tablespoons of the milk and stir until well blended. In a large saucepan, combine the rest of the milk, half-and-half, and butter and bring to a boil, watching carefully to avoid boiling over. Add the cornstarch mixture and continue boiling until thickened.

3. Lower the heat to simmer and add the cheeses. Stir until sauce is smooth. Remove from the heat and quickly stir in each yolk, stirring constantly. Season with salt and pepper.

4. Pour the cheese over the cooked rice elbows and transfer to a well-buttered baking dish. Top with rice bread crumbs, if desired. Bake for 25 minutes, until the top is lightly browned and bubbly.

Angelo Peloni

To Angelo Peloni, the charming Genovese who owns the romantic La Bruschetta restaurant in Los Angeles, risotto is not a dish, it is an act of faith that goes all the way back to Boccaccio. Even though he was raised in Liguria, where string beans, potatoes, and the bold pesto sauces that are this region's signature are more likely to be served on pasta, risotto is something Peloni does by birthright, stirring centuries of tradition with good Arborio rice, which makes the sharing of this treasured family recipe an even larger gift.

Think of risotto as a blank canvas. One night it is studded with sun-dried tomatoes or wild mushrooms, or à la Milanese with saffron and veal marrow, yet another with prosciutto and peas, and on a chilly winter evening, it can be a hearty, soul-satisfying meal with sweet Italian sausage or shrimp and mussels and scallops.

There aren't as many rules for a good risotto as there are variations, but they are important. Always use a wooden spoon. A metal one will ruin the rice and the pot. Always use the best olive oil you can afford or, as Signore Peloni prefers, unsalted butter, *never* margarine. (This dish is about grains of rice, not grams of fat!) Don't skimp on cheese. Buy a good Parmesan or reggiano. Wrapped in cheesecloth, it will keep forever. If time precludes making the beef, chicken, or fish stock yourself, use the best you can find. Always stir it into the risotto warm and keep an extra cup of warm stock on hand, so you don't have to add water if the rice absorbs it too quickly. A good risotto pot is heavy and copper bottomed. If possible, it should have two handles, so you can hang on to it with one hand while you stir with the other, then switch hands.

Risotto requires no special talent, only patience and the ability to daydream and stir at the same time. To enjoy risotto like a true Italian it's important to know that the cognoscenti eat around the edges of the bowl first where the rice cools faster, making a little mound of the rest in the middle of the plate where it will stay hot.

Signore Peloni's secret for the creamiest risotto I have ever tasted is in the final step—whipping the butter, then the cheese, into the dish *before* it is served.

This is your pasta. Learn to do it well.

Risotto Primavera

Serves 4.

¾ cup asparagus spears, sliced in small pieces
1 cup zucchini, sliced and quartered
½ cup frozen peas
½ cup button mushrooms, sliced
1 onion, chopped
1 clove garlic, minced
4 tablespoons (½ stick) butter
1 tablespoon extra virgin olive oil
2 cups Arborio rice
4 cups warm vegetable or chicken stock
½ cup freshly grated Parmesan or reggiano cheese
   Freshly ground pepper
   Salt to taste

1. In a saucepan, parboil the asparagus, zucchini, peas, and mushrooms. Set aside.

2. In a medium saucepan, sauté the onion and garlic with 1 tablespoon butter and the olive oil over low heat. When the onion starts to become translucent, add the rice, stirring with a wooden spoon until it has absorbed all of the butter and oil completely. Add 2½ cups stock, a little at a time, stirring to ensure the rice absorbs all of the liquid completely.

3. Cook for about 15 minutes, then stir in the vegetables. Continue cooking, adding the remaining stock and stirring, for about another 15 minutes, or until the rice is cooked to an al dente consistency. Remove the pan from the heat, add the remaining 3 tablespoons butter, and whip it into the rice to melt it. Add the cheese and whip the rice again. Add salt and pepper to taste.

4. Pour immediately into wide bowls while it is very hot. Grate extra cheese to pass at the table.

Lynn Jamison

Lynn Jamison's tiny bakery and restaurant on Philadelphia's Antiques Row is not one of those pseudo-sophisticated cafés so popular today, all *latte* and relaxation as long as you follow the rules. No, this place, which draws students, struggling artists, antique hunters, and the well-heeled locals out of the historically registered houses that line these streets, feels more permanent than that. The small sunny space recalls the English tea room, the glory days of Greenwich Village, the Left Bank, Mildred Pierce.

The Jamison children rush in and out. The smallest reaches into the showcase for a handful of bear claws and, with sticky fingers, slaps the screen door in his haste to get back to the boys eagerly waiting on the cobblestones for their share. The regulars sit for hours over one of Lynn's extraordinary muffins and the newspaper, a love letter, a poem. No rush. I order the Jax special, my husband the John special, which is anything Lynn feels like making for our breakfast or lunch that day. She knows exactly what is and isn't gluten-free. This is home. My birthday cake comes from here.

Queen Mother Cake

Lynn calls this darkly satisfying chocolate torte Queen Mother Cake, but I think of it as the "mother of all birthday cakes." The recipe here makes two cakes. I always freeze one uniced against the dark day that will need all the sweetening it can get. This is a moist cake, and it will be very wet just after baking. Don't panic. The secret to avoiding collapse is letting it cool completely in the pan.

I serve this cake with a shiny chocolate glaze, but it is equally scrumptious with a thicker frosting, raspberry puree, or even whipped cream. For special occasions, dip jumbo strawberries in extra chocolate glaze and arrange around the top.

Makes 2 9-inch cakes.

CAKE BATTER

      Butter and rice flour for preparing pans
12 ounces bittersweet chocolate
¾ pound (3 sticks) sweet butter

1½ cups sugar
½ teaspoon salt
12 eggs, separated
Pinch cream of tartar
¾ pound finely ground almonds

CHOCOLATE GLAZE AND TOPPING

6 ounces bittersweet chocolate
1½ cups heavy cream
1 cup sliced, unblanched almonds

1. *To make the cake:* Preheat oven to 300°F. Generously butter two round 9-inch cake pans, then dust them well with rice flour.

2. Melt the chocolate in the top of a double boiler, then set it aside and let it cool.

3. In a large bowl, cream the butter, sugar, and salt together. Gently fork-beat the egg yolks, then add to the creamed butter and sugar, mixing thoroughly. Add the cooled chocolate and fold it in.

4. In a separate chilled small bowl, add the cream of tartar to the reserved egg whites and whip into soft peaks. Gently fold the egg whites into the chocolate mixture, then gently fold in the almonds, one-third at a time.

5. Pour into the buttered and floured pans. Bake for approximately 40 minutes, or until a sharp knife inserted comes out almost clean. Cool thoroughly before removing from pans and glazing.

6. *To make the glaze and topping:* Chop the chocolate into small pieces and set aside.

7. In a small saucepan heat the cream to scalding—bubbles should form around the outside edge of the liquid in the pan. Remove the pan from the heat. Mix in the chocolate until it's melted and stir until thick. Let cool. Pour the glaze over the cake and chill thoroughly in the refrigerator.

8. Meanwhile, preheat the oven to 350°F. Sprinkle the sliced almonds on a baking sheet and toast for 7 minutes, watching carefully to make sure they don't burn.

9. When the Queen Mother cake is well chilled and just before serving, sprinkle almonds all over the top.

CHAPTER ELEVEN

Growing Up Wheat- and Gluten-free

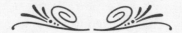

You have to eat oatmeal or you'll dry up. Everybody knows that.

—KAY THOMPSON
from *Eloise*

Children are not so different from you and me. They're really just short grown-ups whose natural tendency to be eccentric has not yet been stifled by rules. Going "against the grain" is as natural to young children as breathing.

Assuming the physical problem has been diagnosed—and that's a big assumption, since a child's symptoms of celiac disease and other grain allergies can be even tougher to pinpoint than an adult's, masquerading as everything from hyperactivity, to growth problems, to listlessness, to attention deficit disorder and requiring round after round of frustrating visits to the doctor—the next step is to ensure compliance, create an atmosphere of normalcy, and plant the seeds of acceptance of this decidedly "uncool" dietary problem.

This is not so easy to do at an age when conformity not only equals acceptance, it is the only requirement in the long climb up childhood's social ladder. Anything that's different is suspect and routinely ridiculed. Those are the rules we all have to live by, and the grain-intolerant child will not be the exception, no matter the danger or the difficulty in getting a wheat- or gluten-free meal. If you persist in drawing the curtain of your own fear around your child, it will be worse.

You may be tempted to rush into every lunch, dinner, sleepover, school trip, picnic, party, and snack situation like the wheat and gluten attack dog you've learned to become, sniffing out every offending crumb before allowing your darling to participate in these food-related activities. This will certainly save your child any accidental exposure to the offending grains, but it can also cause him or her great social angst, shining the spotlight of "special problem" right into his or her embarrassed little face and pushing the envelope of parental paranoia into uncharted territory. Remember how embarrassed you were when your mother made you wear ankle socks with your half-inch heels?

Worry that goes beyond reasonable concern creates another kind of illness. The greatest danger, in my opinion, is raising a child who never grows beyond the narrow definition of special or allergic or intolerant or sick and misses the whole person beyond this restrictive view. We all know adults like this, people who are wounded by their problems instead of challenged by them. They never see themselves as anything but damaged. While no parent can imagine deliberately shaping this neurotic response to life in their own offspring, they can and, unfortunately, do out of the goodness of their intentions.

It may not seem like a big deal, but a good start is refusing to allow your child to be referred to as a "patient." While it is true that your child has an allergy or a disease or an intolerance, illness is no longer present and patient status no longer applies. Unfortunately, children believe what adults say about them. If you don't believe this, reread *The Secret Garden*.

As a parent, it is so easy to be grateful that your child doesn't have a life-threatening illness but a dietary problem that, in your relief, you may overlook the feelings of sadness and loss your child may be experiencing in the wake of diagnosis. These could take the form of antisocial or aggressive behavior, anger, loss of appetite, moodiness, decline in school performance, or even the acquiring of an imaginary friend.

Just as adults experience sadness and loss at the sight of certain foods, often accompanied by feelings of isolation, so too must a child be encouraged to express the grief that inevitably accompanies diagnosis and always turns inward if left unexpressed. I think it's important to create an environment in which a child feels safe enough to talk about this sadness and in which there is no judgment about how it is being expressed. There shouldn't be rules for its expression. If there are, I believe a child quickly gets the message that only the feelings that do not frighten Mommy and Daddy are okay and the ones that do are best left unsaid or dragged out only when we want to scare them.

Try not judge the behavior, but attempt to see what's behind it. Remember that difficult children usually are those who are having difficulties. This rule applies to adults too, who are just larger children with better vocabularies.

This may seem picky, but I don't think a food should ever be labeled "bad." A parent should never say to a small child, "Don't eat that, it's bad for you." It's much healthier for a child to learn to say "No, thank you" to a food, explaining that it does not agree with his or her stomach. This teaches a respect for the differences in people as well as a healthy acceptance for other people's enjoyment of foods that cannot be tolerated personally. It's also a great way to nip in the bud the tendency to blame our problems on external forces, accepting that food is not the villain; our own odd digestive systems are. Food isn't the illness; the illness is.

While this may seem a little too philosophical for a youngster to absorb, consider the alternative: what if you were raised thinking pasta was poison and you discovered you had accidentally eaten a noodle? Perspective is important here. One accident does not death by pasta make. That is your fear, not your child's. You must teach a healthy respect for the repercussions without teaching a person to be afraid to eat.

I'm no Dr. Spock, but I count enough children among my favorite people to know there is a great opportunity here for all parents to teach a definition of special that will carry your little person proudly through any situation life dishes out. The idea is to raise a child who believes everybody wants a bit of *her* sandwich, and not the other way around.

Lots of Don'ts. Some Dos.

Do explain your child's needs to teachers and be careful to explain that celiac disease or food allergy should not exclude your child from participating in anything except standard meals. The idea is to convey the seriousness of the problem without exaggeration, which may cause your child to be treated as an invalid. This is a litigious world, and people may overreact to potential liability if you are not careful to explain that the problem does not extend to activities. People always overreact.

Ditto for consulting with the dietitian who should be key in seeing to it that your child gets a wheat- or gluten-free lunch without undue fanfare, difficulty, or attention. A meeting with the school nurse will alert her if your child is suffering from symptoms. If the occasional or frequent bathroom emergency is still a problem, the person who monitors the passes ought to be alerted ahead of time to save the child embarrassment. I suggest that a signal is agreed upon.

Good parenting is always work. Good parenting of a wheat- or gluten-intolerant child is hard work.

If cookies or other treats are routinely given out, you have to make sure the teacher has a supply on hand for your child, and you have to make sure they are given out without the kind of announcement that will make your little one feel like the class nerd. Comments such as "And what do we have here for little Jaxie Lowell?" are definitely out.

It's important to be very specific with your child's teacher and use examples he or she can understand. Say "You know how you hate it when you're trying to lose forty pounds and you really don't want people to know and a waiter carrying a plate of cottage cheese and lemon wedges shouts, 'Who gets the diet plate?' Well, that's how my son or daughter feels too."

If there's a pizza party, volunteer to make the crusts—there's a great one in this chapter. Give the school dietitian an ample supply of bread, pasta, hamburger buns, and the like. The more the cafeteria is able to treat your child as normal, the more normal your child will feel. If it's a birthday, make the cake. If it's a school outing, volunteer to make one of the dishes.

Some people will be cruel; others will be stupid; and still more will unwittingly try to kill your child with kindness.

Hard as it is to believe, there are parents who will not invite your child to a party because making something special is too much work for them. I met a woman at a Celiac Sprue Association/USA conference whose fourth grader actually was *un*invited when the news of her special requirements reached the insensitive hostess. It is incumbent upon any parent to search these people out and volunteer before they do or say something really stupid and damaging.

There will be grandparents and older friends and relatives who will pooh-pooh the importance of the diet. This is the "in-my-day" crowd. They will tell you to "let him have a little." Do not let them intimidate you. Get them off in a corner and let them know they will not be welcome in your home or you will not return to theirs if this behavior recurs. One parent I know asked if an adult who was told of a child's food intolerance and ignored it is guilty of child abuse. Good question.

Unfortunately, some children with celiac disease do not develop and gain height as easily as other children. While some doctors believe in growth hormones for these small children, I believe that only love can encourage them to be tall inside. Start teaching your child now that stature is never measured in feet and inches.

It's important to involve the whole family. Brothers and sisters should reinforce the importance of their sibling's food and should be encouraged to eat meals that are wheat- and gluten-free. Just because people are small doesn't mean they don't feel just as left out of things as you and I.

Turn the tables and label an entire shelf wheat- or gluten-free. It's nice to own something in this world.

If a child is old enough to read, a child is old enough to read labels. It is never too soon to start taking responsibility.

If it helps everyone rest more easily, a Medic Alert bracelet that says "no wheat" or "no gluten" can be obtained, but frankly, I think this is more for the parent than the child. A bracelet like that is a tough thing to explain in the schoolyard.

Peer pressure doesn't get any easier with age. In fact, it reaches an almost lemminglike stage in adolescence. The son of a friend confided he had a terrible time explaining his celiac disease when all the guys went out for pizza and beer. He told me he felt really "dorky" being the only one who couldn't eat pizza and said he was tempted to forget his diet and run with the pack. I suggested that the truth might be the culprit and advised a cooler explanation than grain intolerance.

"Tell them you're into New Age, macrobiotic, Zen, cruelty-free, politically correct eating." It worked. Brown rice and gluten-free plum balls are now a big thing on campus.

Dating is always an agony even without food. Wheat- and gluten-free dating is hell. How do you tell kids who are sixteen they will be loved for themselves, not their ability to eat hamburgers? The same way you tell them the pimples will go away, the braces will come off, and they should never go out without their rubbers. If you say it enough times, they will believe you and do the right thing.

Enough rules. What's for dinner?

> Some foods make you fat.
> Some foods make you thin.
> Some foods taste so good,
> they just make you want to grin.

There isn't much a kid likes to begin with. Anything green, red, yellow, blue, beige, or gray, fishy, squishy, spicy, smelly, dicey, ricey, gooey, remotely unusual, or not an Oreo cookie is greeted with suspicion, considered "Yuk."

When you consider that the level of dining experience of the average grade schooler is usually limited to cookies and milk, peanut butter and jelly sandwiches, and the occasional reservation at Chuck E. Cheese, you begin to see the special difficulties caused by wheat and gluten intolerance among small children.

In fact, it would not be an exaggeration to say that the smaller the child, the larger the problem. The reason for this is simple. We can and do experiment. They can't or won't, not for at least another fifteen or twenty years.

Compounding the problem is peer pressure—"If I can't have cookies after nap time like everybody else, I'm never going to kindergarten again"—and important philosophical questions, such as "If I can't have birthday cake, will I ever grow up?"

In children's terms, eating well means eating like all the other kids. How would you like to open a lunch box in the middle of the playground and find a bunch of stale rice cakes and an apple, or a rice bread sandwich that tastes like Silly String? Or worse, how would you like to show up at a party and have to sit in the corner because everybody is having pizza but you? This is not a lot of fun for someone who is at the age when conformity equals social acceptance and differences of any kind are tantamount to wetting your pants in fourth grade.

There is quite a bit you can do to ensure your little one not only eats well but eats just like the other kids. If you do it well, one day you may even find your offspring has traded one of your brownies for the latest superhero action figure.

Breakfast

The way to start as we've all been taught, is with a hot breakfast.

> *Pease-porridge hot,*
> *pease-porridge old,*
> *Pease-porridge in the pot,*
> *nine days old.*

Cold rice cereal with bananas, milk, and raisins is always available. There are always wheat- and gluten-free waffles with a little butter and jam. Or some homemade rice bread and peanut butter. Save the following hearty porridge for one of those cold and stormy, yellow-slicker, stick-to-the-ribs kind of days, then head out to wait for the school bus. Double the recipe and send everybody, including yourself, into the world wrapped in a warm hug from home. If time is just too precious for a weekday outing for the whisk, this is a real wintry weekend treat for the whole family. It should go without saying that this is the ideal meal to serve two teddy bears on a picnic.

Who says *Gourmet* magazine is for grown-ups? This wonderful porridge from the March 1991 issue has been reprinted here courtesy of *Gourmet*. Copyright © 1991 by The Conde Nast Publications Inc.

Cornmeal Porridge with Dried Fruit

Serves 2.

2 tablespoons golden raisins
½ cup yellow cornmeal
¼ teaspoon salt
½ cup milk plus additional to pour into cereal
1 tablespoon unsalted butter, halved
8 dried apricots, cut into small pieces
   Light brown sugar or maple syrup

1. In a small bowl, cover the raisins with cold water and let them stand for 10 minutes. In a medium saucepan, whisk together the cornmeal, ½ cup cold water, and the salt until the mixture is smooth. Add 1½ cups boiling water and the ½ cup milk in a slow stream, whisking all the time.

2. Cook the mixture in a double boiler set over a pan of simmering water, stirring often, for 10 to 15 minutes, or until the liquid is absorbed and the porridge is thickened.

3. Divide the porridge between two bowls and top it with the butter, the apricots, and the raisins that have been drained of their water. Serve the porridge with the sugar or maple syrup and the additional milk to taste.

"A Chocolate Chip off the Old Block!"

Everybody has a gluten-free or wheat-free chocolate chip cookie recipe. It doesn't get easier or taste better than this one. It's right from the back of the package of Nestlé Semi-Sweet Chocolate Morsels, and I don't know a child who doesn't gobble them up.

What makes them wheat- and gluten-free is substituting 2¼ cups of packaged wheat- and gluten-free cookie mix (see chapter 4 for your choice of purveyor), which should always be waiting on the shelf, for the 2¼ cups of flour called for in the original recipe. Then add the rest of the ingredients *minus* the baking soda (which should already be in the mix). Take care to use gluten-free vanilla extract or vanilla powder, which is available from Authentic Foods as well as other mail-order companies and should be another pantry item in any home catering to a small sweet tooth.

In eight to ten minutes, you've got a hundred cookies. That may sound like a lot to you, but it isn't when you consider that you've got to make enough for the other kids on the bus trip, so yours doesn't feel nerdy with "special" cookies. After you nibble some yourself, you'll see that's not many at all.

Toll House Cookies Without the Toll

Makes 100 two-inch cookies.

2¼ cups of packaged wheat- and gluten-free cookie mix
       (Check whether it contains baking soda. If not, add
       1 teaspoon baking soda.)
  1 teaspoon salt
  ½ pound (2 sticks) butter, softened
  ¾ cup sugar
  ¾ cup firmly packed brown sugar
  1 teaspoon gluten-free vanilla extract
  2 eggs
  1 12-ounce package (2 cups) Nestlé Semi-Sweet
       Chocolate Morsels
  1 cup chopped walnuts or pecans

1. Preheat the oven to 375°F.

2. In a small bowl, combine the substituted cookie mix and the salt. Set the bowl aside. In a large bowl, cream together the butter, sugar, brown sugar, and gluten-free vanilla until well blended.

3. Beat in the eggs. Gradually add the flour mixture and mix well. Stir in the chocolate morsels and nuts.

4. Drop by rounded teaspoonfuls onto ungreased cookie sheets. Bake for 8 to 10 minutes. Let cool.

As the son of a celiac master chef, Beth Hillson's seven-year-old son has no peer pressure problems at all. He walks into the Hebron Avenue School with a lunch box full of brownies, bagels, sandwiches on homemade white bread, and he's the envy of children born of lesser mortals. He swaggers. He gloats. He's "Kid Cookie." Even the teacher begins to salivate.

Jeremy's Peanut Butter and Jelly Cookies

This Hillson family favorite is adapted from Dorie Greenspan's Sweet Times Cookbook *(William Morrow, 1991), and the chef's secret to these sticky concoctions is making sure everyone gets in on the fun. To make these special cookies really special, let the kids roll the dough into balls, make the indentations, and even fill the centers with jam.*

Makes 4 dozen cookies.

    1 cup rice flour
    ⅓ cup tapioca starch
    ⅓ cup potato starch
    1 teaspoon xanthan gum
    ¾ cup (1½ sticks) unsalted butter, softened
    ½ cup smooth peanut butter
    ½ cup firmly packed light brown sugar
    ¼ cup granulated sugar
    1 teaspoon gluten-free vanilla extract
    2 eggs, separated
    1 cup finely chopped unsalted roasted peanuts
    ½ cup jam or jelly

1. Preheat the oven to 350°F. Lightly oil two cookies sheets or line with parchment paper.
2. In a medium bowl, combine the rice flour, tapioca starch, potato starch, and xanthan gum. Reserve.
3. In a medium bowl, beat together the butter, peanut butter, brown and granulated sugar at medium speed until the mixture is light and fluffy. Add the vanilla and 1 egg yolk, and beat to combine. Add the flour mixture and beat on lowest speed just to combine.
4. In a separate small bowl, beat the 2 egg whites until frothy.
5. Set the peanuts in another small bowl. Lightly flour the hands with additional potato starch, and roll the dough into 1-inch balls.

Roll the balls in the egg whites to coat, and then roll each ball in the chopped nuts.

6. Place the balls on cookie sheets about 2 inches apart and make an indentation in the center of each ball with your pinkie. Fill each indentation with a small amount of jam. Bake 16 to 18 minutes or until golden brown. Cool and store in an airtight container. These may be frozen.

Jim Burns loves the gooey brownies his wife, Barbara, perfected for their son. But why on earth would any self-respecting fifth grader love them too? After all, isn't any food that is not only wheat-free but sugar- and chocolate-free as well yucky?

The Burns are parents. They're smart. So, maybe they fudge the truth a little. Sometimes they forget themselves and compete for the last one of these amazing brownies, but Wiley always wins because that is one of the benefits in being a kid.

Wheat-Free Brownies
(Shhh-don't-tell-Wiley-they're-healthy)

The secret in making these amazingly rich squares is the generous amount of vanilla added to the carob and in using roasted carob powder, never raw. If your child tolerates chocolate well and it is not a philosophical issue at your house, no one will mind if you substitute 2 squares of good, unsweetened chocolate in place of the carob.

Yield: Makes 16 pieces.

    5   tablespoons roasted carob powder or 2 squares
        unsweetened chocolate
  5⅓   tablespoons (⅓ cup) butter
    1   cup honey
    2   eggs
  3–4   tablespoons gluten-free vanilla extract
    ¾   cup oat flour (homemade from 1 cup rolled oats or
        commercial oat flour)
  1½   teaspoons baking powder
    ½   teaspoon salt
    ½   cup walnuts, broken

1. Preheat the oven to 350°F.

2. Melt together the carob powder (or chocolate) and butter in a medium saucepan set over low heat, stirring until thoroughly mixed.

3. Beat together the honey and eggs in a small bowl. Slowly add the carob mixture and beat until blended. Stir in the vanilla.

4. Pulse 1 cup rolled oats in a blender until it turns into flour, about 30 seconds. (Skip this step if you have purchased oat flour.)

5. Sift the flour along with the baking powder and salt into a medium bowl. Add the walnuts. Stir in the carob mixture, using a spatula to blend together. Pour the mixture into a greased 8-inch square baking pan.

6. Bake for 25 minutes. The brownies are done when the mixture is cakelike and pulls in from pan's edge. The center section will be more gooey. Cool 10 to 15 minutes, then cut into squares. If the squares are too soft to cut, refrigerate 15 minutes or more, until firmer.

Pizza! Pizza!

It's impossible to be a normal kid in this world and not eat pizza. It's everywhere there are small fingers leaving cheesy prints on the furniture. It can be the reason more than two kids in one room are called a party. It's why lunchroom microwaves were invented. A candle in it makes it birthday pizza, a pepperoni smiley face can turn any frown upside down, and the smell of one baking can lure a youngster out of any mischief.

Kids don't usually like their toppings as exotic and spicy as grownups, but no matter; what's on it is not as important as having the crusty real thing underneath. Bette Hagman, fiction writer, author of *The Gluten-Free Gourmet* and *More from the Gluten-Free Gourmet* (Henry Holt, 1900, 1993), and a celiac herself, has devoted years of her creative life to the kitchen, testing and developing just the right mix of wheat- and gluten-free flours to duplicate any muffin, scone, bread, cookie, brownie, pie, cake, or biscuit for children of all ages.

She remembers too. Maybe that's why her recipes are so satisfying. There are quite a few sticky imitations out there, but this yeast-rising thick pizza crust is the real thing. This is Bette Hagman's master-piece reprinted from *The Gluten-Free Gourmet*, the home baking bible no wheat- and gluten-free home should be without, with permission from and thanks to our publisher, Henry Holt and Company.

Yeast-Rising Thick Pizza Crust

You don't have to be a kid to love this pizza. This crust freezes well. As long as you're going to the trouble for the kids, make one for yourself with goat cheese, grilled eggplant, sun-dried tomatoes, and basil.

Makes two 12½-inch pizzas. Serves 8 to 12.

> 2 cups rice flour
> 2 cups tapioca flour
> ⅔ cup dry milk powder *or* powdered baby formula (See note.)
> 3½ teaspoons xanthan gum
> 1 teaspoon salt
> 2 yeast cakes, or 2 tablespoon dry yeast granules
> 1 cup lukewarm water, 105 to 115 degrees
> 1 tablespoon sugar
> 3 tablespoons shortening
> ½ cup hot water
> 4 egg whites at room temperature

1. In the bowl of a heavy-duty mixer, put the flours, dry milk, xanthan gum, and salt. Crumble the yeast into the lukewarm water with the tablespoon of sugar added. Melt the shortening in the hot water. With the mixer on low, blend the dry ingredients. Pour in the hot water and shortening, blending to mix. Add the egg whites, blend again, then add the yeast mixture. Beat on high speed for 4 minutes.

2. Spoon half the dough onto a greased cookie sheet or round pizza tin. With your hand in a plastic bag, pat the dough out in a circle about ¼ inch thick except at the edges, which should be higher to contain the sauce and fillings. Repeat with the second half of the dough.

3. Spread immediately with your favorite gluten-free tomato sauce and toppings—shredded mozzarella, jack cheese, salami, sliced green peppers, olives, ground beef, or turkey or pork that has been browned and well cooked in small chunks and drained.

4. There is no need to let this rise, but by allowing 20 minutes of rise time, you will get an even thicker crust. Bake in a preheated 400°F oven for 20 to 22 minutes.

NOTE: If your child has a lactose intolerance as well as one to grain, substitute a corn- or soy-based powdered baby formula for the dry milk powder.

Comfort Food

Sometimes I feel like something smooth and yummy,
something warm and good,
like a hug from Mummy.

Macaroni and cheese really is the ultimate food-really-is-love nursery food. It's rich and velvety and feels so good going down. Imagine never having the memory of such edible cosseting, such pure silken delight. I can't. It would be like having had no childhood at all. We never outgrow its comfort, its soothing slide into our overstressed adult lives, full of worry, sensible salads, and too many cups of coffee, which is why Carrie Bogar created the adult version in chapter 10.

Mmmmmmmmmmacaroni and Cheese

The secret to Chef Bogar's pint-size version of this gratin is the choice of cheeses—the milder the better for still-developing taste buds. Her own Scout loves a mild cheddar in his, but yours may prefer an even milder American. You may want to forget the pepper altogether. I've left it in. It's entirely up to you and your tyke's tolerance for seasoning.

Serves 2 to 4 as a main dish, 4 to 6 as a side dish.

  1   10-ounce box Pastariso elbows, cooked according to package directions
  2   tablespoons cornstarch
1½   cups milk
1½   cups half-and-half
 ¼   pound (1 stick) butter
  4   ounces mild Cheddar cheese
  2   ounces American cheese
  2   ounces cream cheese
  2   egg yolks
 ½   teaspoon salt
 ½   teaspoon coarsely ground black pepper (optional)
  1   or 2 slices brown rice bread crumbed in food processor (optional)

1. Cook the elbows according to package directions until they are al dente. Take care not to overook. Drain and set aside.

2. Preheat the oven to 350°F. Combine the cornstarch with 2 tablespoons milk and stir well, until blended. In a large saucepan, combine the milk, half-and-half, and butter, and bring it to a boil, taking care not to allow the mixture to boil over. Add the cornstarch mixture and continue boiling until thickened. Lower the temperature to simmer and add the cheeses. Stir until the sauce is smooth.

3. Remove the pan from the heat and quickly stir in each yolk, stirring constantly. Season with salt and pepper. Pour the cheese sauce over the cooked rice pasta and pour into a well-buttered baking dish. Top with bread crumbs, if desired. Bake for 24 minutes, until the top is lightly browned and bubbly.

Birthdays

Roses are red
Birthdays are blue
My cake is real chocolate.
I might share it with you.

A child I know once said, "If I can't have a birthday cake, I won't grow up. And if I don't grow up, I'll never get tall. And if I don't get tall, I'll *never* be a ballerina!"

The logic of children is such that no coming of age is complete without this magic celebration food that can make time pass, teeth straight, legs long, and dreams reality. Heavy-tasting substitutes don't count.

Steven Rice, the inventive chef and health guru behind Authentic Foods in Los Angeles, makes a chocolate birthday cake mix that's really worth celebrating. He gets letters all the time from children of all ages who bless him for understanding what it means to be surrounded by smiling faces singing off key and to know the cake that is making its way to your chair, waves of icing shimmering in the candlelight, is blazing just for you. Never mind that he uses maple syrup, not sugar, all natural gluten-free flavorings, and his own bean flour that binds particularly well to most foods, but especially to anything chocolate.

It doesn't get easier making a small birthday person smile than with this chocolate cake mix.

"Authentic" Happy Birthday Cake

Makes 1 single layer cake that serves 12.

2 large eggs
1 cup milk or gluten-free vanilla flavor soy milk
¼ cup corn or safflower oil
1 box of Authentic Foods chocolate cake mix
  (See chapter 3 for mail-order information.)

1. Preheat the oven to 375°F. Place waxed paper on the bottom of a round 8-inch pan and grease lightly with oil.

2. In a medium bowl, mix the eggs, milk, and oil together and beat. Empty the cake mix into a large bowl. Mixing at low speed, slowly add the liquid ingredients to the cake mix, beating until moistened. Then mix at medium speed for 2 minutes.

3. Pour the batter into the pan and bake for approximately 35 minutes, or until a toothpick inserted in the center comes out clean.

4. Allow the cake to cool in the pan for at least 5 minutes, then remove it and place it on a cooling rack. Cool the cake completely before frosting. Ice the cake with your favorite frosting or use the following directions.

NOTE: If you use a round 9-inch pan, reduce the baking time to 30 minutes. For 12 cupcakes, bake approximately 20 minutes.

"Authentic" Sour Cream Ganache

Frosting for 1 cake.

12 ounces bittersweet chocolate
1⅔ cups sour cream

1. In a double boiler melt the chocolate, stirring constantly. Remove the pot from the heat and add the sour cream.

2. Stir the mixture with a rubber spatula until it is uniform in color. Spread the ganache evenly over a cooled cake.

3. Light candles, make wishes, and sing.

CHAPTER TWELVE

The Wheat- and Gluten-free Resource Guide

If it's out there, it's in here.

—NYNEX TELEVISION COMMERCIAL

When I began work on this book, the G & I Kosher Bakery in Flushing, New York, was a bustling business, whipping up gluten-free brownies, chocolate chip loaves, lady fingers, sponge cakes, and old-fashioned bakery cookies and briskly filling orders via the mail, phone, and fax machine.

According to their advertisements, this family bakery survived the ups and downs of business on both sides of the Atlantic for generations, even the severe wheat shortages of World War II Europe when, during a protracted period of scarcity, their founder perfected the art of baking with the only ingredient that was in plentiful supply— potato flour.

I have no idea how the firm ended up in the allergy business, but I like to imagine that years later, when one of the dynasty's sons or daughters went to business school and became a marketing genius and came home and said, "You know, Uncle Moe or Sammy or Saul, you could make a bundle selling this stuff to people who can't eat wheat!" the family discovered its products' untapped potential. I also think that's why the desserts were so good. They were invented for people who still had the taste of wheat very much in their mouths.

229

It doesn't seem fair that people who outsmarted the economic repercussions of an entire world war couldn't make it in the 1990s, but they were no longer there when I last called. I prefer to think of Mr. and Mrs. G and Mr. and Mrs. I as happily retired, on a yacht somewhere in the Mediterranean, tasting the ship's pastry and shaking their heads and saying "In our sleep, we could do better," or in Phoenix, wearing bolo ties and telling funny stories about their escapades in the kitchen. I see them playing the back nine at Pebble Beach before going for a dip in the Pacific. I see them anywhere but out of business involuntarily.

I hope these old friends I have never met have not fallen prey to accident, injury, mayhem, or worse. I don't know where they are today. But I do know I miss them. Life is a little less sweet for their absence.

The following guide lists many of the resources available and open for business at press time. It cannot reflect the moment-by-moment changes in the economic climate or the all-too-inevitable casualties of sudden change in the weather. Nor am I able to guarantee addresses or phone or fax numbers beyond printing. It would be impossible and entirely naive of me to try. On the brighter side, many businesses will open and, it is hoped, remain open long after publication. To those, I say, "Catch you next time."

You should have this book for a long time too—well thumbed, dog-eared, and smudged with a wheat- and gluten-free goody or two, eaten in bed while boning up on your restaurant skills or your midnight mail-order technique. Perhaps you will have even seen the wisdom of buying another copy for those in a position to cook for you— (or hinted that they buy their own)—the sister-in-law who always forgets, the friend who thinks gluten is anything containing glue, your nephew the gastroenterologist so he won't blow the diagnosis for somebody else.

I know we've been taught never to deface a book, especially a hardcover book. In this case, I will forgive you. As new businesses open and others close, pencil in the changes as you discover them— new products, mail-order companies, and family businesses that cater to wheat- and gluten-free diets, either deliberately or unwittingly. This way they'll all be in one place. And if you discover something really great, let me know.

I'll put it in a nice clean edition for you. Next time.

National Associations, Information, Support Groups

American Allergy Association
P.O. Box 640
Menlo Park, CA 94026
(415) 322-1663
Must enclose a self-addressed envelope and two stamps.

American Celiac Society
Dietary Support Coalition
58 Musano Court
West Orange, NJ 07052
(201) 325-8837
Must leave your mailing address.

Canadian Celiac Association
6519-B Mississauga Road
Mississauga, On. L5N 1A6
(905) 567-7195

Celiac Disease Foundation
13251 Ventura Boulevard, Suite 3
Studio City, CA 91604-1838
(818) 990-2354
FAX (818) 990-2379

Celiac Sprue Association (CSA)/
   USA
P.O. Box 31700
Omaha, NE 68131-0700
(402) 558-0600

The Gluten Intolerance Group of
   North America, Inc.
P.O. Box 23053
Seattle, WA 98102-0353
(206) 325-6980
(GIG does not have local affiliates, but will gladly supply the names and numbers of support groups in your area.)

Local American Celiac Society Support Groups, CSA/USA Chapters, GIG-recommended Groups, and Independent Support Groups

ARKANSAS

CSA Arkansas/Ozark Celiac
   Support Group
For information: Marilyn H.
   Jorgensen, (501) 492-5243

ARIZONA

CSA Tucson
For information: Pat Ewing,
   (602) 297-1834
CSA Sunshine Chapter
For information: Russ Boocock,
   (602) 837-1953

CALIFORNIA

CSA Orange County
For information: Cecile Weed,
   (714) 750-9543

CSA Redlands Area Celiac
   Support Group
For information: Patricia Siddel,
   (909) 793-3712

CSA Sacramento, California/
   Sprue & You
Information for adults: Susan K.
   Miguel (Sacramento)
Kathe G. Hughes (Stockton),
   (916) 726-3850
Information for children: Kathy B.
   Samuel, (609) 931-5113

CSA San Diego
For information: Lisa A. McPhee,
   (619) 451-3452

CSA Sonoma County Celiac
For information: Laura
   Southworth, (714) 798-3112

COLORADO

CSA Denver/Metro Area Chapter
For information: Betty Elofson,
   (303) 238-5145

CSA Pikes Peak
For information: Virginia Ludwig,
   (719) 598-6748

CONNECTICUT

CSA Celiac Support Group of
   Northwest Connecticut
For information: Marilyn Duffany,
   (203) 283-8506

CSA Connecticut/Nutmeg
   Chapter
For information: Jennifer
   Masterson, (203) 743-5127

CSA Greater Hartford Area
   Chapter
For information: Kathleen Bosse,
   (203) 688-4162

FLORIDA

Celiacs of Orlando, Florida
For information: Mike Jones,
   (407) 856-3754

The Celiac Support Group of
   N.W. Florida/Mary Ester
For information: June Lawrie,
   (904) 581-0807

Crystal River, Florida Celiacs
For information: Mary Lou
   Thomas, (904) 795-7987

CSA Southeast Florida Celiac
   Support Group
For information: Vincent A. Tria,
   (305) 447-1065

The Gluten Intolerance Group of
   Florida
For information: Mary Alice
   Warren, (407) 784-5696

Sarasota, Florida, Celiacs
For information: Sandy Sroufe,
   (813) 921-3701

Tallahassee, Florida, Celiacs
For information: Irma Bass-Paul,
   (904) 562-4177

Tampa Area Celiacs
For information: Candi Rowen,
   (813) 961-0992

GEORGIA

Smyrna/CSA Atlantic Celiac
   Sprue Support Group
For information: Jan Austin,
   (404) 433-9661

ILLINOIS

CSA Central Illinois Celiacs
For information: Marsha Bishoff,
   (309) 444-7415

CSA Greater Chicago Area
   Chapter
For information: Gladys Johnson
   (708) 834-5797

CSA Rockford Area Chapter
For information: Jolyn M. Fasula,
   (815) 877-5302

INDIANA

CSA Indiana Gluten Intolerance
Support Team
For information: Nancy H.
Linnemann, (317) 497-0665

CSA Indianapolis Celiac Sprue
Support Group
For information: Terri Rehm,
(317) 842-8969

IOWA

CSA Waverly Chapter
For information: Betty Bast,
(319) 352-4740

KANSAS

CSA Topeka Celiac Sprue Support
Group
For information: Andrea Clark,
(913) 266-2625

CSA Wichita Celiacs
For information: Kay Finn,
(316) 686-7034

LOUISIANA

Baton Rouge Area CSA Celiac
Support Group
For information: Glenda Worm,
(504) 751-7980

MARYLAND

CSA Maryland Chapter
(C.A.T.C.H.)
For information: Elli Waite
or Marian Wilmoth,
(410) 574-5371
or Mary Humphries
(410) 433-5249

MASSACHUSETTS

Boston Area Support Group
For information: Marina Keegan,
(508) 358-2416

MICHIGAN

CSA Mid-Michigan Chapter
For information: Donovan J.
Sprick, (313) 733-6857

CSA Tri-County Celiacs
For information: Kathy Davis,
(313) 332-2938

MINNESOTA

CSA Midwest Gluten Intolerance
Group
For information: Lois Robertson,
(612) 925-6136

MISSOURI

CSA Greater Kansas City Chapter
For information: Dean Cling,
(816) 942-6677

CSA St. Louis Chapter
For information: Joan Fitzsimmon,
(314) 351-5114

MISSISSIPPI

CSA Gulf Coast Celiac Sprue
Support Group
For information: Jane Dacey,
(601) 875-2820

NEBRASKA

CSA Midlands Chapter
For information: Sandra Allen,
(402) 468-5386

Lincoln/CSA Star City Area
  Chapter
For information: Ruby Bacon,
  (402) 464-4757

NEW JERSEY

American Celiac Society/Mid-
  New Jersey Support Group
For information: Diane Paley,
  (908) 679-6566

American Celiac Society/Southern
  New Jersey Support Group
For information: Christine Kucma,
  (609) 953-1691

CSA Support Group of Central
  New Jersey
For information: Diane Eve Paley,
  (908) 679-6566

NEW MEXICO

Albuquerque/CSA Gluten
  Intolerance Support Group
For information: Marilyn Johnson,
  (505) 299-5283

NEW YORK

American Celiac Society/Capital
  District Celiac Support Group
  (Albany)
For information: Julie Lasky,
  (518) 869-2436

CSA Long Island Celiacs
For information: James J.
  Callahan, (516) 794-1654

CSA New York/Staten Island
  Celiac Society
For information: Lila T. Barbes,
  (718) 984-8547

CSA West New York GF Diet
  Support Group
East Aurora, NY
For information: Joanne
  Hameister, (716) 655-0849

NORTH CAROLINA

CSA North Carolina Celiacs
For information: Ruth Thomas or
  Susan Black, (910) 875-3186

NORTH DAKOTA

CSA North Dakota Celiacs
For information: Juli Becker,
  (701) 742-2738

OHIO

CSA Greater Cleveland Celiacs
For information: David C. Tabar,
  (216) 835-9110

OKLAHOMA

CSA Oklahoma CS Support
  Group
For information: Winnolia
  Porterfield, (405) 942-3818

PENNSYLVANIA

CSA Greater Pittsburg Area CS
  Support Group
For information: Maureen Perkey,
  (412) 922-0295

Greater Philadelphia Celiac Sprue
  Flourtown, PA Support Group
For information: Phyllis Brogdon,
  (215) 836-7518

RHODE ISLAND

CSA Rhode Island CS Support
  Group
For information: Rosalie Jalbert,
  (401) 823-5585

TEXAS

CSA Houston Celiac Sprue
  Support Group
For information: Janet Rinehart,
  (713) 783-7608

CSA San Antonio Celiac Sprue
  Support Group
For information: William Mickish,
  (210) 341-4218

CSA West Texas GF Awareness
  Group
For information: Pat Gatlin,
  (915) 563-4847

Ft. Worth/CSA Lone Star Celiac
  Support Group
For information: Tad Taylor,
  (817) 595-5305

WASHINGTON, D.C.

CSA Celiac Sprue Support Group
For information: Caroline Wolf
  Harlow, (202) 462-8988

WISCONSIN

CSA Fox Valley Celiacs
For information: Joyce Kiekhaefer,
  (414) 734-7695

CSA Madison Area Gluten
  Intolerance Group
For information: Margret
  Siedschlag, (608) 238-3321

CSA Milwaukee Sprue Crew
For information: Luanne Williams,
  (414) 453-4319

Professional and Lay Associations, Government Agencies, Diagnostic Clinics, Information, Referrals, and Research

The American Academy of
  Allergy & Immunology
Allergy information referral line:
  (800) 822-2762

American Board of Medical
  Specialties
Doctor's Credentials/Board
  Certification
  (800) 776-CERT

American Board of Pediatrics
NCNB Plaza, Suite 402
1436 East Rosemary Street
Chapel Hill, NC 27514
(919) 929-0461

American Digestive Disease
  Society
420 Lexington Avenue
New York, NY 10017
(212) 687-3088

American Gastroenterological
  Association
6900 Grove Road
Thorofare, NJ 08086
(609) 848-1000

Celiac Disease Clinic
University of California
San Diego Campus at La Jolla
9500 Gilman Drive, La Jolla, CA
   92093
Dr. Kagnoff or Dr. Anders Nyberg
(619) 534-4622

The Center for Genetics,
   Nutrition and Health
Suite 530 S Street, NW
Washington, DC 20009
(202) 462-5062

Coalition of Digestive Disease
   Organizations
295 Madison Avenue
New York, NY 10017
(212) 685-3440

Food Allergy Network
4744 Holly Avenue
Fairfax, VA 22030
Information, referrals, support for
   wheat-free living:
(703) 691-3179

Food and Drug Administration
Consumer Inquiries
(301) 443-3170

Food and Drug Administration
Med Watch
(800) FDA-1088
All adverse reactions to medical
products (such as medication that
is labeled gluten-free and causes
problems) should be reported
here.

Internal Revenue Service
Washington, DC 20402
Taxpayer Information
(800) 829-1040

LAC/USC Medical Center
Rancho Los Amigos Medical
   Center, Dept. of Pediatrics
7601 East Imperial Highway
Downey, CA 90242
(310) 940-7847
Comprehensive clinical,
   diagnostic, and research

National Center for Nutrition and
   Dietetics of the American
   Dietetic Association
216 West Jackson Boulevard
Chicago, IL 60606-6995
(312) 899-4853
FAX (312) 899-1739
To contact a registered dietitian in
   your area, call:
Consumer Nutrition Hot Line
(800) 366-1655 9 A.M. to 4 P.M.
   EST Monday–Friday

National Digestive Diseases
   Information Clearing House
P.O. Box NDDIC
Bethesda, MD 20892
(301) 468-6344

National Institute for Health
Genetic, Immunologic and
   Gastroenterological Research
(301) 496-4000

The North American Society for
   Pediatric Gastroenterology
69 Butler Street, S.E.
Atlanta, GA 30303

UMAB/Bressler Research Building
Pediatric GI & Nutrition
   Laboratory
655 West Baltimore Street,
   Room 10-047
Baltimore, MD 21201

Dr. Karoly Horvath
(410) 706-1997
Antigliadin IgA and IgG and
antiendomysial antibody tests
for celiac disease

University of Iowa Foundation for
Celiac Disease Research
The University of Iowa Hospital &
Clinics
Department of Internal Medicine
200 Hawkins Drive
Iowa City, IA 52242
Dr. Joseph Murray
(319) 356-8246

University of Maryland's
Department of Pediatric
Gastroenterology and Nutrition
22 South Green Street, Room
N5-W70
Baltimore, MD 21201
Dr. Alessio Fasano
(410) 328-0812
Blood tests for celiac disease. Will
not take patients over 21 years
of age.

U.S. Department of Agriculture
Washington, DC 20402
(800) 535-4555

On-line Computer Services

COOKING/NUTRITION/SPECIAL
DIET INFORMATION

America Online: (800) 827-6364
CompuServe: (800) 848-8199
Genie: (800) 638-9636
Prodigy: (800) 776-3449

Equipment

BREAD MACHINES

For information on all models,
suggested retail price, and
distributors:

Hitachi Home Bakery Breadmaster
(800) 241-6558, Ext. 720

Maxim (Accu-Bakery)
(800) 233-9054

Mister Loaf Home Bakery
(800) 858-3277

National Bread Bakery
(717) 373-7757

Panasonic Bread Bakery
(714) 373-7282

Regal Kitchen Pro
(414) 626-2121

Toastmaster Bread Box
(800) 947-3744

Trillium Breadman
(800) 800-8455

Williams-Sonoma Bread Baker
(800) 541-2233

Welbilt (Homemade Bakery, The
Bread Machine, The Bread
Maker, The Bread Oven)
(516) 365-5040 Ext. 321
Welbilt's new bread machine with
a 1-pound capacity is designed
especially for celiacs and is
available October 1994.

Zojirushi Home Baker
(800) 733-6270

Drugs

For information and ingredients
on over-the-counter and
prescription medications:

A. H. Robins Company
1405 Cummings Drive
Richmond, VA 23220
(800) 762-4672

Bristol-Myers Products/Squibb
345 Park Avenue
New York, NY 10154
(800) 722-9292

Burroughs Wellcome Company
3030 Cornwallis Road
Research Triangle Park, NC 27709
(800) 722-9292

CIBA-Geigy Consumer
   Pharmaceuticals
Mack Woodbridge II
581 Main Street
Woodbridge, NJ 07095
(800) 452-0051

Fisons Consumer Health
Rochester, NY 14623
(800) 334-6433

Glenbrook Laboratories
(Division of Sterling Drug
   Company)
90 Park Avenue
New York, NY 10016
(800) 331-4536

Johnson & Johnson—Mark
   McNeil/PPC, Inc.
Fort Washington, PA 19034
(215) 233-7700

Lakeside Pharmaceuticals
(Division of Merrill Dow)
2110 East Galbraith Road
Cincinnati, OH 45215
(800) 453-4865

Lederle Labs
679 Route 46
Clifton, NJ
(800) 282-8805

Luden's Inc.
(Division of Hershey Foods)
Hershey, PA 17033
(800) 486-1714

Merrill Dow
P.O. Box 1467
Pittsburgh, PA 15230
(800) 453-4865

Miles, Inc.
3040 Windsor Court
Elkhard, IN 46514
(800) 800-4793

Parke-Davis/Warner-Lambert
Morris Plains, NJ 07950
(800) 524-2624

Richardson-Vicks
(Proctor & Gamble)
P.O. Box 599
Cincinnati, OH 45201
(800) 843-9657

Rhone-Poulenc/Rorer
   Pharmaceuticals, Inc.
Fort Washington, PA 19034
(800) 548-3708

Sandoz Pharmaceutical Corp.
East Hanover, NJ 07936
(800) 453-5330

Schering-Plough
Memphis, TN 38151
(901) 320-2011

SmithKline Beecham Corp.
One Franklin Plaza, Philadelphia
 PA 19103
(800) 245-1040

Upjohn
7000 Portage Road
Kalamazoo, MI 49001
(800) 253-8600

Whitehall Labs
685 Third Avenue
New York, NY 10017
(800) 322-3129

Food Companies

For questions, verification,
information on ingredients,
stabilizers, fillers, flavorings, and
the like, contact:

American Home Products
685 Third Avenue
New York, NY 10017
(212) 878-5000

Beatrice Foods
(800) 228-0159

Ben & Jerry's Homemade
Consumer Affairs
P.O. Box 240
Waterbury, VT 05676
(802) 244-6957

Best Foods Baking Group
(Arnold, Brownberry, Thomas)
100 Passaic Avenue
Fairfield, NJ 07004
(800) 356-3314

Betty Crocker Foods
Box 1113
Minneapolis, MN 55440
Desserts, potatoes, convenience
 foods: (800) 328-6787
Snacks: (800) 231-0308
Cereal: (800) 328-1144

Borden
180 East Broad Street
Columbus, OH 43215
(614) 225-4511 (collect calls
 accepted)

Bush Brothers & Company
Bush's Best Baked Beans
P.O. Box 52330, Dept. C
Knoxville, TN 37950

Campbell Soup Company
(Campbell, Franco-American, V-8,
 Swanson, Prego, Pepperidge
 Farm, Vlasic, Marie's, Mrs.
 Paul's, Godiva)
1 Campbell Place,
Camden, NJ 08103-1701
(609) 342-4800
Campbell's Kid Collection:
 (800) 243-4769
Product Inquiries: (800) 770-5858
 or (800) 257-8443

ConAgra Frozen Foods
(Armour, Banquet, Butterball
 Turkey, La Choy, Morton,
 Rosarita, Swift-Eckrich)
Box 3768
Omaha, NE 68103
(800) 722-1344

Continental Baking Company
Checkerboard Square
St. Louis, MO 63164
(800) 222-7575

Dannon Co. Inc.
P.O. Box 44235
Jacksonville, FL 32231
(800) 321-2174

Jimmy Dean Foods
8000 Centerview Parkway
Suite 400
Cordova, TN 38018
(800) 543-4859

Dole Packaged Goods
5795 Lindero Canyon Road
Box 1-55
Westlake Village, CA 91362
(800) 232-8888

Durkee Foods
Pleasanton, CA
(800) 843-8686

General Foods
(Jell-O Pudding and Pie Fillings)
(800) 431-1001

Gooch Foods
(La Rosa, Russo, Budget Pasta)
Box 80808
Lincoln, NB 68501
(800) 228-4060

Gorton Foods
128 Rogers Street
Gloucester, ME 01930
(800) 225-0572

Häagen-Dazs Co. Inc.
Consumer Relations
P.O. Box 550
Minneapolis, MN 55440
(800) 767-0120

Healthy Choice
ConAgra Frozen Foods
Box 3768
Omaha, NE 68103
(800) 323-9980

H. J. Heinz
1062 Progress Street
Pittsburgh, PA 15212
Consumer Affairs USA:
   (412) 237-5740

Hershey Foods
Consumer Relations, 100 Crystal
   A Drive
Hershey, PA 17033
(800) 468-1714

Hillshire Farms & Kahn's
3241 Spring Grove Avenue
Cincinnati, OH 45225
(800) 543-8615

Hunt-Wesson Foods
Hunt Wesson, Inc.
Box 4800
Fullerton, CA 92634
(714) 680-1431 (collect calls
   accepted)

Hygrade Food Products
40 Oak Hollow Road, Suite 355
Southfield, MI 48034
(800) 782-5486

Kellogg Company
Box CAMB
Battle Creek, MI 49016
(800) 962-1413
For allergy-related questions:
   (800) 962-1718

Kraft/General Foods
Glenview, IL 60025
(800) 634-1984
For cereal information:
   (800) 431-POST

Nabisco Foods
East Hanover, NJ 07936
(800) 932-7800

Newman's Own
(Salad dressings, sauces, popcorn)
Westport, CT 06880
(203) 222-0136

Ore-Ida Foods
Box 10
Boise, ID 83707
(208) 383-6800

Oscar Mayer
(800) 222-2323

Pillsbury
Box 550
Minneapolis, MN 55440
(800) 767-4466

Quaker Oats Company
P.O. Box 049003
Chicago, IL 60604
(800) 494-7843

Sara Lee Bakery Products
224 S. Michigan Avenue
Chicago, IL 60604
(800) 323-7117

The J. M. Smucker Company
Orrville, OH 44667
(216) 682-0015

Starkist Foods
One Riverfront Place
Newport, KY 41071
(800) 252-7033

TCBY
(800) 876-TCBY

Van Den Bergh Foods
(Ragu and Chicken Tonight
   Sauces)
Lisle, IL 60532
(800) 328-7248

Yoplait USA
Box 1113
Minneapolis, MN 55440
(800) 967-5248

Baby Foods

Beech-Nut
Research & Development
Box 618
St. Louis, MO 63188
(800) 523-6633

Gerber Foods
Gerber Products
Fremont, MI 49413
(800) 4-GERBER

Heinz Foods
General Office
Box 57
Pittsburgh, PA 15230
(800) 872-2229

Toothpastes, Powders, Mouth Washes, Rinses

Arm & Hammer
(800) 624-2889

Chesebrough Ponds
(800) 786-5135

Colgate Palmolive
300 Park Avenue, New York, NY
   10022
(800) 221-4607

The Procter & Gamble Company
6071 Center Hill Road
Cincinnati, OH 45224
(800) 543-7270

Not-to-Miss Health Food Stores on a Supermarket Scale

Fresh Fields
4948 Boiling Brook Parkway
Rockville, MD 20852
For locations of stores in the
Washington, DC, Philadelphia,
Chicago, and New York
metropolitan areas . . .
(301) 984-3737

Whole Foods Market, Inc.
601 North Lamar
Suite 300
Austin, TX 78703
For locations of Whole Foods
Markets in Texas, Louisiana,
Northern California, Michigan,
and in the Chicago metropolitan
area . . .
Bread & Circus Markets in Rhode
    Island and Boston . . .
Wellspring Grocery in North
    Carolina and Mrs. Gooch's in
    Los Angeles . . .
(512) 328-7541 or (312) 587-9760

Health Food and Specialty Store Foods

Abraham's Natural Foods
(Wheat-free sweet rice cookies)
Long Branch, NJ 07740

Alta Dena Certified Dairy
(Alta Dena Natural Ice Cream and
    Frozen Desserts)
City of Industry, CA 91744
(Each container bears plant
    number for referrals.)

Anne Lanyi Foods
(Salad dressings)
P.O. Box 2032
S. Londonderry, VT 05155
(Write for recipes/gluten-free
    varieties.)

Arrowhead Mills
(Gluten-free flours and mixes)
P.O. Box 2059
Hereford, Texas 79045

Barbara's Pinta Chips
(Salsa and pinto bean chips)
Barbara's Bakery, Inc.
3900 Cypress Drive
Petaluma, CA 94954
(707) 765-2273

Blanchard & Blanchard Spa
    Dressings
Norwich, VT 05055
(800) 334-0268

Bob's Red Mill Natural Foods, Inc.
(Gluten-free flours)
5209 S.E. International Way
Milwaukie, OR 97222
(503) 654-3215 or (503) 653-1339

Cascadian Farm
(Frozen desserts)
P.O. Box 218
Tualatin, OR 97062

Cedarlane Natural Foods
(Gluten-free lasagne and wheat-
    free macaroni and cheese)
1864 East 22 Street
Los Angeles, CA 90058

Cooks Flavoring Co.
(Gluten-free extracts)
3319 Pacific Avenue
Tacoma, WA 98408
(206) 727-1361

David's Goodbatter
(Organic wheat- and gluten-free
  pancake and baking mixes)
Box 102
Bausman, PA 17504
(717) 293-7833

DeBoles Nutritional Foods
(Corn pastas)
2120 Jericho Turnpike
Garden City, NY 11040
(516) 742-1818

Edward & Sons
(Brown rice snaps)
Edward & Sons Trading Company
P.O. Box 1326
Carpinteria, CA 93014
(805) 684-8500

Enrico's Ketchup
Ventre Packing Co. Inc.
6050 Court Street Road
Syracuse, New York 13206
(315) 463-2384

Erewhon
(Wheat and gluten-free cereals)
U.S. Mills
4301 North 30th Street
Omaha, NE 68111
(402) 451-4567

Fantastic Foods
(Wheat- and gluten-free soup
  mixes)
1250 North McDowell Boulevard
Petaluma, CA 94954

Foods by George
(Distributed by Shiloh Farms)
(Wheat- and gluten-free ravioli
  and pastas)
108 Schimmel Street
Paramus, NJ 07652
(201) 265-8167

Fran's Fresh Foods
(Wheat-free baked goods)
161 White Horse Pike
Waterford Plaza
Atco, NJ 08004
(800) 331-DIET

Glenn Foods
(Glenny's Brown Rice Treat—
  wheat-free)
999 Central Avenue
Woodmere, NY 11598

Gold Mine Natural Food
  Company
(Ohsawa Wheat-free soy and
  tamari sauces)
San Diego, CA 92102
(800) 475-3663

Grainaissance, Inc.
(Mochi)
1580 62nd Street
Emeryville, CA 94608
(510) 547-7256

Guiltless Gourmet Inc.
(Fat-free dips and no-oil tortilla
  chips)
3709 Promontory Point Drive
Austin, TX 78744
(800) 723-9541

Hain Pure Food Company, Inc.
50 Charles Lindbergh Blvd.
Uniondale, NY 11553
(800) 434-4246

Health Valley Foods
(Soups, chili, and other canned
  foods)
16100 Foothill Boulevard
Irwindale, CA 91706
(800) 423-4846

Imagine Foods, Inc.
(Rice Dream soy milk and
  nondairy frozen desserts)
350 Cambridge Avenue, Suite 350
Palo Alto, CA 94306

Integrity Baking Company
(Wheatless maple walnut cookies)
R.D. #3, Box 788
Franklinville, NJ 08322
(609) 694-4235

Lady J. Inc.
(Original Lady J wheat-free
  cookies)
P.O. Box 1307
Menlo Park, CA 94025
(415) 329-0588

Michele Martin Desserts
(Healthy Munchies individually
  packaged wheat-free cookies)
201 Greenfield Avenue
Ardmore, PA 19003
(610) 896-7320

Millina's Finest
(Pasta sauces)
Organic Food Products, Inc.
P.O. Box 1510
Freedom, CA 95019

Mitoku Co. Ltd.
(Mitoku Macrobiotic wheat-free
  soy sauce)
Tokyo, Japan 100

Mrs. Denson's Cookie Co. Inc.
(Mrs. Denson's Wheat-free
  cookies)
9651 Highway 101 North
Redwood, CA 95470

Mr. Spice Sauces
(Exotic sauces, gluten wheat,
  dairy, salt, fat, and cholesterol-
  free)
711 Namquid Drive
Warwick, RI 02888
(800) SAUCE 4U

Mrs. Leeper's, Inc.
(Wheat and gluten-free corn and
  rice pastas)
11035 Technology Place, #300
San Diego, CA 92127
(619) 673-0073

Muir Glen Inc.
(Organic Chef Sauces)
424 North 7th Street
Sacramento, CA 95814
(800) 832-6345

Mystic lake Dairy, Inc.
(Yeast-, wheat-, and gluten-free
  bread)
24200 N.E. 14th Street
Redmond, WA 98053
(206) 868-2029

Nature's Warehouse
(Wheat-free packaged cookies)
P.O. Box 161525
Sacramento, CA 95816

Northern Soy Inc.
(Soy Boy Not Dogs—vegetarian
  hot hogs)
545 West Avenue
Rochester, NY 14611

Omega Nutrition
(Wheat- and gluten-free almond
  and hazelnut flours)
6505 Aldridge Road
Bellinham, WA 98226
(604) 622-8862 or
(800) 661-3529

Nature's Hilights
(Rice crust pizza)
P.O. Box 3526, Chico, CA 95927
(800) 313-6454

Pacific Grain Products
(Wheat- and gluten-free rice
crackers and snacks)
P.O. Box 2060
Woodland, CA 95776
(916) 662-5056

Pamela's Products, Inc.
(Wheat- and gluten-free cookies)
156 Utah Avenue
South San Francisco, CA 94080
(415) 952-4546

Pastariso Products, Inc.
(Wheat- and gluten-free rice
pastas)
55 Ironside Crescent, Unit 6 & 7
Scarborough, Ont.
Canada M1X 1N3
(416) 321-9090

Pocono Heart of Buckwheat
Pocono Buckwheat Cookbook
P.O. Box 440 PC
Penn Yan, NY 14527
(Write for recipe booklet.)

Quinoa Corp.
American Quinoa Harvest
(Wheat-free cereals)
P.O. Box 1039
Torrance, CA 90505
(310) 530-8666

Red Mill Farms
(Wheat- and gluten-free cakes and
cookies)
290 South 5th Street
Brooklyn, NY 11211
(718) 384-2150

Shelton's Poultry, Inc.
(Wheat- and gluten-free chicken
and turkey franks, lunch meats,
and poultry products)
204 North Loranne Avenue
Pomona, CA 91767

Shiloh Farms, Inc.
(Wheat- and gluten-free baking
mixes)
Sulphur Springs, AR 72768

Stonyfield Farm
(Natural yogurts and nonfat
frozen yogurt)
10 Burton Avenue
Londonderry, NH 03053

Terra Chips
(Spiced sweet potato and mixed
exotic vegetable chips)
Dana Alexander, Inc.
39 Norman Avenue
Brooklyn, NY 11222

Tree of Life
(Wheat-free tamari sauce)
P.O. Box 410
St. Augustine, FL 32084
(904) 824-1846

Tumaro's
(Frozen black bean enchiladas)
5300 Santa Monica Boulevard,
Suite B 16
Los Angeles, CA 90029
(213) 464-6317

Turtle Mountain, Inc.
(Sweet Nothings nondairy frozen
desserts)
P.O. Box 70
Junction City, OR 97448
(800) 859-SAVE

One percent of profits donated to save the sea turtles.

21st Century Foods
(Masa)
30A Germania Street
Jamaica Plain, MA 02130
(617) 522-7595

Uncle Dave's Kitchen
(Uncle Dave's natural pasta
   sauces)
Route 30, P.O. Box 69
Bondville, VT 05340
(802) 297-0008

Van's International Foods
(Wheat- and gluten-free pancakes
   and waffles)
1751 West Torrance Boulevard,
   Unit K
Torrance, CA 90501
(310) 320-8611

Vitasoy USA, Inc.
(Lactose-free flavored soy milks)
Box 552
Busbani, CA 94005

Vita Spelt Products
(Spelt pasta products for wheat-
   free but not gluten-free diets)
Purity Foods
2871 West Jolly Road
Okemos, MI 48864

WestBrae Natural
(Wheat- and gluten-free crackers
   and snacks)
Pacific Grain Products
Woodland, CA 95776
(916) 662-5056

Mail-order Foods

See also chapter 4 for comprehensive list and reviews.

Ellef's Gluten-Free
(Baked goods, baking mixes, pizza
   crusts)
M.P.O. Box 2703
Niagara Falls, NY 14302
(416) 562-3086 or
3866 23rd Street
Vineland, Ont.
Canada LOR 2CO

Fiddler's Green Farm
(Wheat-free pancake and baking
   mixes)
RR 1, Box 656
Belfast, ME 04915
(207) 338-3568

Hearty Mix
(Gluten-free mixes)
1231 Madison Hill Road
Rahway, NJ 07065
(908) 382-3010

The Karlich Company
(Foods free of common allergies)
(305) 474-9612

Life Source Natural Food Limited
91 Esna Park Drive
Markham, Ont.
Canada L3R 2S2
(905) 831-5433

Miss Roben's Dietary Foods
(Gluten-free mixes and baking
   items)
P.O. Box 1434
Frederick, MD 21702
(800) 891-0083

Natural Feast Corporation
(Wheat- and gluten-free fresh fruit
  pies)
P.O. Box 4200
Peabody, MA 01961

Old Windmill Specialty Foods
(Wheat- and gluten-free baked
  goods and mixes)
5014 16th Avenue, Suite 202
Brooklyn, NY 11204
(800) 653-3791
Fax (718) 633-8980

Special Foods
(Wheat-free breads and mixes
  from unusual flours)
9207 Shotgun Court
Springfield, VA 22153
(703) 644-0991

Sterk's Bakery
(Wheat- and gluten-free breads,
  cakes, cookies)
1402 Pine Avenue, Suite 543
Niagara Falls, NY 14031
(800) 608-4501 or
3866 23rd Street
Vineland, Ontario, Canada LOR
  2CO
TEL/FAX: (905) 562-3086

**Restaurant Chains, Fast Food
Restaurants, Ice Cream and
Frozen Yogurt Stores**

Arby's
Box 407008
Ft. Lauderdale, FL 33340
(305) 351-5110

Baskin-Robbins
31 Baskin-Robbins Place
Glendale, CA 91201
Consumer Affairs: (800) 331-0031

Ben & Jerry's Homemade
P.O. Box 240
Waterbury, VT 05676
Consumer Affairs: (802) 244-6957

Boston Chicken
Consumer Response Team
1804 Centre Point Drive
P.O. Box 3117
Naperville, IL 60566
(800) 365-7000

Burger King
17777 Old Cutler Road
Miami, FL 33157
(800) YES-1800

Carvel Corporation
Ft. Lauderdale, FL 33340
(800) 322-4848

Chi-Chi's
Box 32338
Louisville, KY 40232
(502) 426-3900

Chuck E. Cheese
4441 West Airport Freeway
Irving, TX 75062
(214) 258-8507

Columbo Yogurt
Frozen Products Division
5 Branch Street
Methuen, MA 01844
(800) 221-5431

Denny's
203 East Main Street
Spartanburg, SC 29319
(803) 597-7396

Friendly's
1855 Boston Road
Wilbrahma, MA 01095
(413) 543-2400

Häagen-Dazs Co. Inc.
Glenpoint Centre East
Teaneck, NJ 07666
(800) 767-0120

Hardee's
1233 Hardees Boulevard
Rocky Mount, SC 27804
(800) 777-8000

International House of Pancakes
525 North Brand Boulevard
Glendale, CA 91203
(818) 240-6055

KFC/Kentucky Fried Chicken
For information: (800) CALL KFC

McDonald's
One Kroc Drive
Oak Brook, IL 60521
(708) 575-6198

McDonald's Corporation
Nutrition Information Center
One Kroc Drive
Oak Brook, IL 60521
(708) 575-FOOD

Olive Garden
Guest Relations
5900 Lake Ellenor Drive
Orlando, FL 32809
(800) 331-2729

Outback Steakhouse
550 North Reo Street
Tampa, FL 33609
(813) 282-1225

Ponderosa Steakhouse
S & A Restaurant Corp.
12404 Park Central
Dallas, TX 75251
(214) 404-5000

Red Lobster
Guest Relations
Box 593330
Orlando, FL 32859

Roy Rogers
Consumer Affairs: (410) 859-8618

Shoney's
171 Elm Hill Pike
Nashville, TN 3702
(615) 391-5201

Sizzler International
12655 West Jefferson Boulevard
Los Angeles, CA 90066
(310) 827-2300

Subway
325 Bic Drive
Milford, CT 06460
(800) 888-4848

Taco Bell
1701 Von Karman
Irvine, CA 92714
(800) TAC-OBEL

TCBY
1100 TCBY Tower
425 West Capitol Avenue
Little Rock, AR 72201
(501) 688-8229 or (800) 876-
   TCBY

Wendy's
(800) 443-7266

Travel

See also chapter 7 for information on trains, planes, and boats.

INFORMATION AND REFERENCE MATERIAL

Fairchild Travel Industry Personnel Directory
Fairchild Books
(800) 247-6622

Health Information for International Travel
Superintendent of Documents
U.S. Government Printing Office
Washington, D.C. 20402
(202) 783-3238

The Travel Guide to Gluten Free Foods Across Canada
Canadian Celiac Association/
   L'Association Canadienne
   de la Maladie Coelique
(416) 567-7195

RAILROADS NOT DISCUSSED IN CHAPTER 7

Austrian Rail (212) 944-6880

Brit Rail (212) 575-2667

DER Tour/German Railway (800) 421-2929

Japan Railways (212) 332-8686

Rail Europe (800) 4-EURAIL

South American Princess Rail Tours (800) 835-8907

TRAVEL AND TOUR COMPANIES

Abercrombie & Kent (800) 323-7308

Maupintour (800) 255-4260

Travel Agents International (800) 242-4242

American Youth Hostels and
   Hostelling International
733 15th Street NW, Suite 840
Washington, DC 20005
(202) 783-6161 FAX (202) 783-6171

Spa Finders
91 Fifth Avenue
New York, NY 10003
(800) 255-7727

International Celiac Societies and Associations

FOR SHOPPING, DINING, AND OTHER USEFUL TRAVEL INFORMATION

Please Note: When calling the following countries (except Canada) from the United States, dial 011 or seek assistance from the overseas operator. When dialing these numbers from within each country, eliminate the country code (usually the first one, two, or three digits) and apply local calling instructions, as codes vary from country to country.) Some overseas phone numbers are unavailable. Please make note of these addresses and write well in advance of travel to insure assistance.

ARGENTINA

Asistencia al Celiaco de la
  Argentina
Casila de Correo 5555
1000 Buenos Aires
Republica Argentina
Contact: Mrs. Alicia Greco
Telex: 17354 Inserar
Fax (541) 331-3863

Asociacion Celiaca Argentina—
  Sede Central
Calle 2 No 1578, e/64 y 65
1900 La Plata
Buenos Aires
Republica Argentina
Phone: 54-21-31320/31030
Fax 54-21-210288/30907

Asociacion Pro Ayuda Al Celiaco
Personeria Juridica 212 "A"
CC567—Coreo Central—5000
  Cba
Cordoba
Republica Argentina

AUSTRALIA

The Coeliac Society of New
  South Wales
P.O. Box 271
Wahroonga 2076, New South
  Wales, Australia
Contact: Cheryl Price
Phone: 612/498/2593

The Coeliac Society of South
  Australia
106A Hampstead Road
Broadview 5083, South Australia,
  Australia
Contact: Harry Dunn
Phone: 61/8/266/3899

The Coeliac Society of Western
  Australia
P.O. Box 219
Mount Lawley 6050
Western Australia, Australia
Contact: Jane Mikus
Phone: 61/9/337/3504

The Queensland Coeliac Society
P.O. Box 530
Indooroopilly 4068
Queensland, Australia
Contact: John Nichols
Phone: 61/7/378/5747

The Victorian Coeliac Society
P.O. Box 22
Chadstone Centre 3148
Victoria, Australia
Contact: Jan Parker
Phone: 61/3/772/7086

Western Australia Takes Care of
  Tasmanian Coeliacs
18 Garfield Street
Launceton 7250
Tasmania, Australia
Contact: Jenny Tilley
Phone: 61/03/446653

AUSTRIA

Oesterreichische
  Arbeitsgemeinschaft Zoliakie
Anton-Baumgartner-Strasse 44/C5/
  2302
A-1232 Wien, Austria
Contact: Hertna Deutsch
Phone: 43/1/6708523

BELGIUM

S.B.M.C.—B.C.V.
International Contacts
A 20 Ave. L. Bertrand 100
B - 1030 Brussels, Belgium
Contact: F. Vander Linden
Phone: 32/2/216/8347 Fax:
   32/2/216/8347

Vlaamse Coeliakievereniging
Ter Weibrock 29
B-9880 Aalter, Belgium
Contact: Jose Deguffroy
Phone: 32/1/74/28/45

BULGARIA

Bulgarian Coeliac Society
Pl. Slavieikov 9
Sofia 1000, Bulgaria
Contact: Isadors Zaidner

CANADA

Canadian Celiac Association
(See listing on page 231.)
Contact: Mrs. Rosie Wartecker
Phone: 1/416/567/7191
Fax: 1/416/567/7191

DENMARK

Dansk Coliaki Forening
Bellisvej 31
DK-3650 Olstykke, Denmark
Contact: C. C. Brandt-Pedersen
Phone: 45/4217/4664 Summer: 45/
   9733/8345

EGYPT

World Health Organization
P.O. Box 1517
Alexandria 21511, Egypt
Contact: Dr. M. H. Wahdan

ESTONIA

Tartu University
Int. Medical Clinic
Ulikooli 18
Tartu EE 2400, Estonia
Contact: Prof. V. Salupere

FAROE ISLANDS

Coliaki Felag Foroya
FR-510 Nordragote
Faroe Islands
Contact: Mrs. Marita Olsen
Phone: 298/4/16/71

FINLAND

Suomen Keliakiayhdistys R.Y.
Toolonkatu 56 A5
SF-00250 Helsinki, Finland
Phone: 358/90/440745

FRANCE

Association Francaise des
   Intolerants au Gluten
89 Rue du Faubourg Saint Antoine
F-75011 Paris, France
Contact: Mme. Gabrielle Cambus
Phone: 33/1/43/47/0447

GERMANY

Deutsche Zoliakie-Gesellschaft
   e.V.
Filderhaupstrabe 61
Stuttgart 70, Germany
Phone: 33/711/454514
Fax: 49/711/4567817

GREECE

Hellenic Coeliac Society
125 Ippokratous Street
GR-Athens 114 72, Greece
Contact: Mr. P. Plessas
Phone: 30/136/14/366 or 30/1/46/
   18/081

HUNGARY

Liszterzekenyek
   Erdekkpviseletenek
Orszagos Egyesulete
Palanta U. 11
H-1025 Budapest, Hungary
Contact: Mrs. Tunde Koltai
Phone: 36/1/202/7396 & 6892 or
   36/1/135/1278
Fax: 36/1/155/9816

ICELAND

Samtok Folks med Glutenopol
Logafold 15
IS-112 Reykjavik, Iceland
Contact: Mr. Magnus Asgeirsson
Phone: 354/675064
Fax: 354/603350

IRELAND

The Coeliac Society of Ireland
Carmichael House
4 North Brunswick Street
Dublin 4, Ireland
Phone: 353/1/31478

ISRAEL

The Israel Coeliac Society
Rehov Rabinowitz 9
ISR—96549 Jerusalem, Israel
Phone: 972/2/412635

ITALY

Associazione Celiachia Palermo
Casella Postale No. 1
Succursale No. 42
I-90124 Palermo, Italy
Contact: Lo Bue Domenica

Associazione Famiglie Bambini
   Celiachi
Via Masia 21
I-40138 Bologna, Italy
Contact: Emilia Romague
Phone: 39/51/391980

Associazione Italiana per la
   Celiachia
Via Picotti, 22
I-56100 Pisa, Italy
Contact: Signora Annamaria
   Vallesi Sereni
Phone: 39/50/580939

Italian Coeliac Association
Piazza Costituzione Italiana, 2
I-50063 Figline Valdarno
Firenze, Italy
Contact: Sr. Adriano Pucci
Phone: 39/55/959680 or 39/55/
  9509575

MALTA

Coeliac Association
"Lumet"
Upper Gardens
St. Julians STJ 05, Malta
Contact: Mrs. Mary Rose Caruana
Phone: 35/370778

THE NETHERLANDS

Nederlandse Coeliakie Vereniging
Deimos 5
NL—3402 JG IJsselstein, The
  Netherlands
Contact: Alice van der Wal-
  Dekker

NEW ZEALAND

Coeliac Society of New Zealand
18 Rutherford Terrace
Meadowbank
Auckland 5, New Zealand
Contact: Margaret Ashcroft

NORWAY

Norsk Coliaki Forening
Prinsens Gate 6.5. etg.
N-0152 Oslo, Norway
Phone: 47/22/42/60/01 (Tuesday
  and Wednesday)
Fax: 47/22/42/60/04

POLAND

T.P.D.
U1. Jasna 24/26
PL-00-950 Warszawa, Poland
Contact: Magdalena Loska
Phone: 48/22/27/78/44

PORTUGAL

Clube dos Coliacos
Pediatria Hosp. Santa Maria
P-1600 Lisboa, Portugal
Phone: 351/749327

ROMANIA

Aglutena
Sdr. Avram lanca nr 24
2400 Sibiu, Romania
Contact: Karin Kober
Phone: 417622 or 433050 Ext.
  268

SLOVENIA

Slovensko Drustvo za Celiakijo
Ljubljanska 5
62000 Maribor, Slovenia
Contact: Breda Kojc

SOUTH AFRICA

Coeliac Society of South Africa
91 Third Avenue
Percelia 2192
Johannesburg, South Africa
Contact: Mrs. M. Kaplan
Phone: 27/440/3431

SPAIN

A.C.E. Delegaacion Comtabria
Apdo. Correos 291
E-39080 Santander Spain
Contact: Emmique Cueto
Phone: 34/33/63/85

A.C.M. Asociacion de Celiacos de
  Madrid
C/Pozas, 4-Local
E-28004—Madrid, Spain
Contact: Manuela Marquez
Phone: 34/1/523/04/94

E.Z.E. Asociacion Celiaca de
  Euzkadi
Somera. 3-3o-Dpto 2
E-48005 Bilbao, Spain
Contact: Mireia Apraiz
Phone: 34/4/416/94/80
S.M.A.P. Celiacs de Catalunya
Ronda Universidad No. 21—80-F
E-08007 Barcelona Spain
Contact: Madilde Torralba
Phone: 34/317/72/00 Ext. 98

SWEDEN

Svenska Celiakiforbundet
Box 9040
S-102 71 Stockholm, Sweden
Contact: Bjorn Johansson
Phone: 46/669/86/72 Fax: 46/668/
  74/05

SWITZERLAND

Associacion Romande de la
  Coeliakie
2 Avenue Agassiz

CH-1001 Lausanne, Switzerland
Contact: M J-F Tosetti
Phone: 021/319/71/11 Fax: 021/
  319/79/10

Gruppo della Svizzera Italiana
  degli Interessati al Problema
  della Celiachia
Fam. E + S Pedrazzoli
Contrada Isolabella 1, Pedevilla
Ch-6512 Giubiasco, Switzerland
Phone: 41/92/27/34/54

Schweizerische
  Interessengemeinschaft fur
  Zoliakie
Schaulistrasse 4
CH-4142 Munchenstein,
  Switzerland
Phone: 41/61/46/21/87

UNITED KINGDOM

The Coeliac Society of the United
  Kingdom
P.O. Box No 220
High Wycombe, Bucks
HP11 2HY, England, U.K.
Contact: Mrs. J. Austin
Phone: 44/494/437278
Fax: 44/494/474349

URUGUAY

Asociacion Celiaca del Uruguay
  ACELU
Charrua 2318
Montevideo, Uruguay
Contact: Sra. Ana. Ma Grassi de
  Monteverde

Required Reading

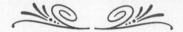

Newsletters

Celiac Disease Foundation
  Newsletter
13251 Ventura Boulevard, Suite 3
Studio City, CA 91604
(818) 990-2354
Fax: (818) 990-2379

The Gluten-Free Baker Newsletter
Editor/Baker Sandra J. Leonard
361 Cherrywood Drive
Fairborn, OH 45324
(513) 878-3221

Gluten-Free Living
P.O. Box 105
Hastings-On-Hudson, NY 10706

Lifeline
Newsletter of the Celiac Sprue
  Association/USA
P.O. Box 31700
Omaha, NB 68131
(402) 558-0600

Reference

All About Food Allergy by Faye M.
  Dong (George F. Stickley Co.,
  1984)

The Allergy Self Help Book by Sharon
  Faelton & *Prevention Magazine*
  (Rodale Press, 1983)

*The Complete Guide to Anti-Aging
  Nutrients* by Sheldon Saul
  Hendler (Simon & Schuster,
  1985)

*The Complete Guide to Food Allergy and
  Intolerance* by Dr. Jonathan
  Brostoff and Linda Gamlin
  (Crown, 1989)

*Food Finds, America's Best Local Foods
  and the People Who Produce Them*
  by Allison and Margaret Engel
  (HarperCollins, 1991)

Gluten Intolerance by Merri Lou
Dobler (American Dietetic
Association, 1991) (Call 800-
745-0775 to order.)

*Grossman's Guide to Wines, Spirits and
Beers* (Charles Scribner's Sons,
1983)

Healing Nutrients by Patrick Quillin
(Contemporary Books, 1987)

*Hugh Johnson's Modern Encyclopedia of
Wine* (Simon & Schuster, 1991)

*Larousse Gastronomique, The
Encyclopedia of Food, Wine &
Cookery* by Prosper Montagne
(Crown, 1961)

Let's Eat Right to Keep Fit and *Let's Get
Well* by Adelle Davis (New
American Library, 1954, 1965)

*The Merck Manual of Diagnosis and
Therapy,* Published by Merck
Sharp & Dohme Research
Laboratories

Natural Healing by Mark Bricklin
(Rodale Press, 1983)

The Physicians' Desk Reference
(Medical Economics Data,
yearly)

Prescription drug and over-the-
counter editions
P.O. Box 10689
Des Moines, IA 50336
(515) 284-6782
FAX (515) 284-6714

Cooking and Baking

The Allergy Self Help Cookbook by
Marjorie Hurt Jones, RN
(Wings Books, 1984)

The Art of Mexican Cooking by Diana
Kennedy (Bantam, 1989)

*The Carolina Rice Kitchen: The African
Connection* by Karen Hess
(University of South Carolina
Press, 1992)

Coping with the Gluten-Free Diet by
Marion Wood (Charles C.
Thomas, 1982)

Delicious and Easy Rice Flour Recipes
by Marion Wood (Charles C.
Thomas, 1981)

Essentials of Classic Italian Cooking by
Marcella Hazan (Knopf, 1993)

The Foods & Wines of Spain by
Penelope Casas (Alfred A.
Knopf, 1982)

"Full of Beans" Low-fat, high-fiber,
heart-healthy recipes
Published by the Canadian
Celiac Association/L'Association
Canadienne de la Maladie
Coelique (416) 567-7195

The Gluten-Free Gourmet by Bette
Hagman (Henry Holt, 1990)

Gluten Intolerance Group Cookbook by
Elaine Harstook (Gluten
Intolerance Group, 1990)

Gourmet Food on a Wheat Free Diet by
Marion Wood (Charles C.
Thomas, 1979)

*In Praise of the Potato: Recipes from
Around the World* by Lindsey
Bareham (Penguin, 1993)

Mesa Mexicana by Mary Sue Milliken and Susan Feniger with Helene Siegal (William Morrow, 1994)

Modern Southwest Cuisine by John Rivera Sedlar (reissued by Ten Speed Press, 1994)

More from the Gluten-Free Gourmet by Bette Hagman (Henry Holt, 1993)

The New Laurel's Kitchen by Laurel Robertson, Carol Flinders and Brian Ruppenthal (Ten Speed Press, 1986)

A Passion for Potatoes by Lydie Marshall (HarperCollins, 1992)

The Rice Book by Sri Owen (St. Martin's Press, 1994)

Rice, The Amazing Grain by Marie Simmons (Henry Holt, 1991)

Riso—Undiscovered Rice Dishes of Northern Italy by Gioietta Vitale with Lisa Lawley (Crown, 1992)

Risotto, A Taste of Milan by Constance Arkin Del Nero and Rosario Del Nero (Harper & Row, 1988)

Sheila Lukins's All Around the World Cookbook (Workman Publishing, 1994)

On the Internet

If you have a computer modem, you can join a free celiac dis-

cussion group being formed on the Internet.

Open and unmoderated, the discussion list will include the latest scientific research (written for the layperson) as well as information on which foods are gluten free and which are not and how to cope with such issues as the developmental delays and changes sometimes brought on or aggravated by gluten (autism, attention deficit disorder, and others). Users will also find recipes and cooking tips, advice on finding gluten-free food by mail order, and information on eating out safely.

To subscribe, send the following command in the BODY of email to LISTSERV @SJUVM.STJOHNS.EDU on the Internet: SUB CELIAC yourfirstname yourlastname. For example: SUB CELIAC John Doe

If you have any problems, contact one of the list owners: Michael Jones celiac@ispace.com at (407) 856-3754. If you call, please do so during business hours. No commercial advertisements are allowed on this list.

IMPORTANT: In the spirit of open exchange, this list is unmoderated; anyone can post to it. Therefore, it is possible that the information in it may not be accurate. Users must draw their own conclusions about how to use the information on this list. The list owners strongly suggest that users do their own analyses of any claims made.

Appendix

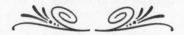

The "Photocopy-and-Pack" wheat allergy and gluten intolerance explanation cards I've created—with a lot of help from my friends—are a fast and easy way of getting around eating wheat and gluten while you're getting around the world. Appearing below in English and translated into French, Spanish, Italian, German, Portuguese, Swedish, Danish, Hebrew, Russian, Greek, Polish, Japanese, and Chinese, on the following pages, the cards should let any waiter or chef, provided that he or she can read (I'm not being rude here—some can't), know at a glance which foods are off-limits to you.

Before you head off for parts unknown, just make several copies of the appropriate card and stick them in your luggage, your purse, your passport, between the pages of your favorite guide book, even in your camera case. Once abroad, present a copy to your waiter, but with a smile. And remember, using someone's native tongue, even if it's written down, is a lot more polite than pointing or trying to be understood by yelling louder and louder in English.

WHEAT ALLERGY CARD

I do not speak your language.

I'm allergic to wheat and all its derivatives.

If I eat any food, product, chemical additive, or stabilizer containing even a trace of this grain, I will become ill.

If necessary, please check with the chef to make sure my food does not contain any of the ingredients listed above and help me order a meal I can safely enjoy.

Thank you very much!

GLUTEN INTOLERANCE CARD

I do not speak your language.

I have celiac disease.

If I eat any food, product, chemical additive, or stabilizer containing even a trace of wheat, rye, oats, buckwheat, barley, millet, triticale, grain vinegar, malt, or any derivatives of these grains, I will become ill.

I am able to eat foods containing corn and rice.

If necessary, please check with the chef to make sure my food does not contain any of the ingredients listed above and help me order a meal I can safely enjoy.

Thank you very much!

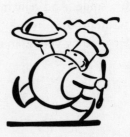

WHEAT ALLERGY CARD

Je ne parle pas votre langue.

Je suis allergique au blé et ses extraits.

Si je mange n'importe quel genre de nourriture, produit, engrais chimiques ou préserve contenant même une trace de ce graine, je tomberai malade.

Si possible, veuillez avertir le chef cuisinier d'être sûr que ma nourriture ne contient pas les engraís que je viens de mentioner et de m'aider à choisir un repas que je pourrai savourer sans inquiétude.

Merci beaucoup.

GLUTEN INTOLERANCE CARD

Je ne parle pas votre langue.

J'ai une malade intestinale.

Si je mange n'importe quel genre de nourriture, produit, engrais chimiques ou préserve contenant même une trace de blé, seigle, sarrazin, orge, millet, tritacole, graine, vinaigre, malte ou les extraits de ses graines, je tomberai malade.

Je peut manger de la nourriture à base de mais et riz. Si possible, veuillez avertir le chef cuisinier d'être sûr que ma nourriture ne contient pas les engraís que je viens de mentioner et de m'aider à choisir un repas que je pourrai savourer sans inquiétude.

Merci beaucoup.

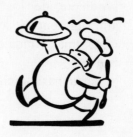

Spanish

WHEAT ALLERGY CARD

No hablo su idioma.

Soy alérgico al trigo y sus derivados.

Si como cualquier comida, producto, aditivo químico o establzador que contenga este grano, me voy a enfermar.

Si es necesario, por favor averigue con el cocinero para asegurarse que mi comida no contenga ninguno de los ingredientes antes mencionados y ayúdeme a ordenar una comida que pueda disfrutar.

¡Muchas Gracias!

GLUTEN INTOLERANCE CARD

No hablo su idioma.

Sufro de Infantilismo Intestinal (Enfermedad Celiaca)

Por lo cual no puedo comer ningún alimento, producto, aditivo químico o establzador que contenga trigo, centeno, avena, trigo, sarraceno, cebada, mijo, "tritacale", vinagre de grano, malta, o ninguno de los derivados de estos granos sin enfermarme.

Peudo comer cualquier alimento que contenga maíz y arroz.

Si es necesario, por favor averigue con el cocinero para asegurarse que mi comida no contenga ningún ingrediente de los especificados anteriormente y ayúdeme a ordenar una comida que pueda disfrutar.

¡Muchas Gracias!

Italian

WHEAT ALLERGY CARD

Non parlo Italiano.

Sono allergico al grano e a tutti i suoi derivati.

Se mangio cibi che contengono prodotti o derivati di grano, anche in quantita minima, mi sento molto male.

Per favore mi aiuti a ordinare un buon pasto che non includa grano o derivati di grano.

Se e necessario per favore si consulti con il cuoco.
Grazie.

GLUTEN INTOLERANCE CARD

Non parlo Italiano.

Sono affetta dal morbo Celiaco.

Se mangio del cibo contenente prodotti o solo tracce di grano, avena, segala, orzo, crusca, malto e aceto digrano, mi sento molto male.

Posso pero mangiare cibi che contengono riso e granturco.

Se e necessario si consulti con il cuoco per assicurarsi che il mio cibo non contenga nessuno dei prodotti sopra elencati e mi aiuti a scegliere un buon pasto.

Grazie.

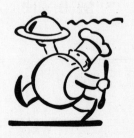

German

WHEAT ALLERGY CARD

Ich spreche kein Deutsch.

Ich habe eine Allergie gegen den Weizen und seine Ableitungen.

Wenn ich esse etwas Speise, Erzeugnis, Zusatz oder Stabilisator mit gerade eine Spur von Weizen, dann ich werde krank.

Im Notfall, bitte den Küchenchef um Hilfe bitten dass meine Speise erhält kein Weizen und daher ich kann mit Sicherheit essen.

Danke schön.

GLUTEN INTOLERANCE CARD

Ich spreche kein Deutsch.

Ich habe eine Krankheit.

Wenn ich esse etwas Speise, Erzeugnis, Zusatz oder Stabilisator mit gerade eine Spur von Weizen, Roggen, Hafern, Buchweizen, Gerste, Hirse, Malz, Getreideessig oder andere Ableitungen von deiser Getreiden, dann ich werde krank.

Können Sie bitte den Küchenchef meine Probleme erklären so dass meine Speise erhält keine Bestandteile, wie hinoben verzeichnen sind, und geben Sie mir Hilfe um ein Gericht dass ich darf mit Sicherheit essen zu bestellen.

Danke schön.

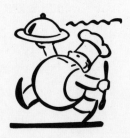

Portuguese

WHEAT ALLERGY CARD

Eu não falo a sua lingua.

Eu sou alérgica ao trigo e a todos os seus derivados.

Se eu como qualquer alimento ou estiver em contato com qualquer um desses grãos fico doente.

Por favor se necessário verifique com o chefe de cozinha para ter certeza que meu prato nao tenha esses ingredientes. Eu realmente apreciaria se voce pudesse me ajudar com a minha escolha.

Muito obrigada.

GLUTEN INTOLERANCE CARD

Me desculpe, mas eu não falo o português.

Por sofrer de um tipo de doenca intestinal, eu nao posso comer nenhum alimento ou estar em contato com produtos ou aditivos quimicos que contenham: trigo, centeio, aveia, trigo sarraceno, cevada, malte ou qualquer derivados desses grãos, sendo que se o fizer, eu fico doente.

Eu sei que posso comer milho e arroz.

Por favor cheque se necessário com o cozinheiro para que nenhum dos pratos tenham esses ingredientes.

E eu realmente apreciaria se voce pudesse me ajudar a escholher um prato que eu possa comer sem perigo.

Muito obrigada.

Polish

WHEAT ALLERGY CARD

Nie władam twoim językiem.

Mam alergię na pszenicę i jej pochodne.

Jeżeli zjem jakiekolwiek pożywienie, środki kons-erwujące czy wyrób zawierający nawet śladowe ilości pszenicy, rozchoruję się.

Proszę pomóc mi wybrać posiłek, który nie zagra-żałby memu zdrowiu, jak również, jeżeli jest to konie-czne, proszę upewnić się u szefa kuchni, że moje jedzenie nie zawiera żadnego z powyższych skład-ników.

Bardzo dziękuję.

GLUTEN INTOLERANCE CARD

Nie władam twoim językiem.

Choruję na celiaklię (zaburzenia wchłaniania z jelit).

Jeżeli zjem jakiekolwiek pożywienie, środki kons-erwujące czy wyrób zawierający nawet śladowe ilości pszenicy, żyta, owsa, gryki, jęczmienia (pęczak, kasza perłowa), prosa, octu zbożowego, słodu, czy jakich-kolwiek pochodnych tych zbóż, rozchoruję się.

Mogę za to jeść pożywienie zawierające kukury-dzę lub ryż.

Proszę pomóc mi wybrać posiłek, który nie zagra-żałby memu zdrowiu, jak rów-nież, jeżeli jest to konieczne, proszę upewnić się u szefa kuchni, że moje jedzenie nie za-wiera żadnego z powyższych składników.

Bardzo dziękuję.

Swedish

WHEAT ALLERGY CARD

Jag talar inte svenska.

Jag är allergisk mot vete i alla dess former.

Om jag äter någon som helst mat, produkt, kemisk tillsats eller stabiliseringsämne som innehåller bara en aning av vete så kommer jag att insjukna.

Var vänlig kontrollera med Er kock att min mat inte innehåller någon av ingredienserna enligt ovan.

Jag uppskattar att Ni hjälper mig att beställa rätter som jag kan njuta av i säker förvissning om att inte insjukna.

Tack så mycket!

GLUTEN INTOLERANCE CARD

Jag talar inte svenska.

Jag lider av Celiaki (dvs glutenintolerans).

Om jag äter någon som helst mat, produkt, kemisk tillsats eller stabiliseringsämne som innehåller bara en aning av vete, råg, havre, bovete, korn, hirs, triticale (en korsning mellan durumvete och råg), vinäger (baserad på dessa produkter) eller malt så kommer jag att insjukna.

Jag kan äta mat som innehåller majs eller ris.

Var vänlig kontrollera med Er kock att min mat inte innehåller någon av ingredienserna enligt ovan.

Jag uppskattar att Ni hjälper mig att beställa rätter som jag kan njuta av i säker förvissning om att inte insjukna.

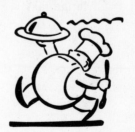

Tack så mycket!

WHEAT ALLERGY CARD

Jeg taler ikke Dansk.

Jeg er allergisk mod hvede i alle former.

Hvis jeg spiser nogen som helst mad, produkt, kemisk tilsaettelse eller stabiliserande emne sä bliver jeg meget syg.

Vil De vaere venlig at kontrollere med kokken at min mad ikke indehälder noget som helst af de hvede produkter jeg har naevnt og vil de ogsä hjaelpe mig med at bestille et mältid som jag kan nyde uden risiko forat blive syg.

Mange tak!

GLUTEN INTOLERANCE CARD

Jeg taler ikke Dansk.

Jeg lider af Glute-intolerance.

Hvis jeg spiser nogen som helst mad, produkt, kemisk tilsaettelse eller stabiliserande emne som indeholder kun en smule hvede, rug havre, byg, hirse, gaerengs eddike eller malt sä bliver jeg meget syg.

Jeg kan spise mad som indeholder majs og ris.

Vil de vare vaenlig at kontrollere så min mad ikke indeholder nogen af de ovenfor naevnte ingredienser.

Vil de vare vaenlig at hjaelpe mig med at bestille et mältid som jeg kan nyde uden risiko for at blive syg.

Mange tak!

Hebrew

WHEAT ALLERGY CARD

אני לא מדבר את השפה שלכם.
יש לי אלרגיה לחיטה ולכל מה שנגזר ממנה.
אם אני אוכל מאכל כלשהו, מוצר, תוספת כימית או
מָנַצָב שיש בו גרעך זה, אני אחלָה.
אם יש צורן, אנא תבדוק עם הטבח כדי לאשר שבאוכל
שלי איך אף אחד מהמרכיבים הנייל ובבקשה תעזור
לי להזמיך משהי שאוכל להנות עם בטחון.
תודה רבה.

GLUTEN INTOLERANCE CARD

אני לא מדבר את השפה שלכם.
יש לימחלה 'מֶלִיאַקְ'.
אם אני אוכל מאכלכלשהו, מוצר, תוספת כימית או
מיצב שיש בו אפ׳לו טיפה: חיטה, שיפוך, שיבולת-שועל,
חיטה מוסלמית, שעורה דוחך, 'טְרִיטָקַאל', חמץ
של גרעיך, לֶתֶת או כל מוצר שנגזר מהנ״ל,
אני אחלָה.
אני יכול לאכול כל דבר שעשוי מתירס ואורז.
אם יש צורן, אנא תבדוק עם הטבח כדי לאשר שבאוכל
שלי איך אף אחד מהמרכיבים הנ׳׳ לובבקשה תעזור לי
להזמיך משהו שאוכל להנות עם בטחוך.
תודה רבה.

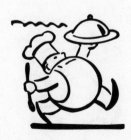

WHEAT ALLERGY CARD

Я не говорю на вашем языке.

У меня аллергия на пшеницу и все её производные.

Мне противопоказаны продукты питания, химические добавки или стабилизаторы, содержащие даже минимальное количество пшеницы.

Если необходимо, пожалуйста свяжитесь с шеф-поваром с тем, чтобы удостовериться, что моя пища не содержит перечисленных выше ингридентов. Помогите мне заказать блюдо, которое я смогу безопасно есть.

Большое спасибо!

GLUTEN INTOLERANCE CARD

Я не говорю на вашем языке.

У меня заболевание органов брюшной полости.

Моему организму противопоказаны продукты питания, химические добавки или стабилизаторы, содержащие даже минимальное количество пшеницы ржи, овсянки, гречихи, ячменя, проса, зернового уксуса, солода, или их производных.

Я могу потреблять продукты из кукурузы и риса.

Если необходимо, пожалуйста дайте знать шеф-повару, что моя пища не должна содержать никаких из перечисленных выше ингридентов и помогите мне заказать блюдо, которое я смогу безопасно есть.

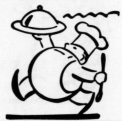

Большое спасибо!

Greek

WHEAT ALLERGY CARD

Δέν μιλώ την γλώσσα σας

έχω αλλεργία στο σιτάρι και σε όλα τα παράγωγά του.

Εάν φάω οποιοδήποτε φαγητό, προιόν, χημικό πρόσθετο ή σταθεροποιητή που περιέχει έστω και ίχνη αυτού του σπόρου, θά αρρωστήσω.

Αν είναι αναγκαίο, παρακαλώ επικοινωνήστε μέ τόν Σέφ ώστε να αποκλεισθεί κάθε πιθανότητα τό φαγητό μου νά περιέχει οποιοδήποτε από τα παρα πάνω συστατικά καί για να με βοηθήσει να παραγγείλω ένα φαγητό χωρίς να ανησυχώ.

Σας ευχαριστώ πολύ.

GLUTEN INTOLERANCE CARD

Δέν μιλώ την γλώσσα σας

Πάσχω από εντερική νόσο.

Εάν φάω οποιοδήποτε φαγητό, προιόν ή χημικό πρόσθετο ή σταθεροποιητή που περιέχει ακόμη και ίχνη σιταριριού, σίκαλης, βρώμης, κριθαριού, κέχρου, ξυδιού ή τριταδε ? ή οποιοδήποτε παράγωγο αυτών των σπόρων θά αρρωστήσω.

Μπορώ νά τραφώ μέ φαγητά που περιέχουν καλαμπόκι και ρύζι.

Αν είναι αναγκαίο, παρακαλώ επικοινωνείστε . . .

WHEAT ALLERGY CARD

#1 小麦

1. 私は貴方の國の言葉を話しません。
2. 私はの小麦およびそれを原料とするすべての製品に対してアレルキーがあります。
3. もし、小麦の粉が少しでも含まれた食品、製品、化學薬品、あるいは安定剤を口にすれば、私は病気になつてしまいます。
4. もし、その恐れがあるようでしたら、私の食事に上記の原料が含まれていないことを、どうか料理長に確認をして下さい。私が何の心配もなく食事ができるように、注文の手助けをして下さい。
5. 御協力をありがとうごさいます。

GLUTEN INTOLERANCE CARD

#2 グルテン

1. 私は貴方の國の言葉を話しません。
2. 私は小児脂肪便症です。
3. もし、小麦、ライ麦、からす麦、そぽ、大麦、きぴ、トリタケール、穀物酒、麦芽酒（モルツ）、あるいはこれらの粉を原料とするいかなる食品、製品、化學薬品、安定剤でもひとたび口にすれば、私は病気になつてしまいます。
4. 私は、とうもろこしや米でできた食品を摂つてもかまいません。
5. もし、その恐れがあようでしたら、私の食事に上記の原料が含まれていないことを、どうか料理長に確認をして下さい。私が何の心配もなく食事ができるように、注文の手助けをして下さい。
6. 御協力をありがとうごさいます。

Chinese

WHEAT ALLERGY CARD

小 麦

我不懂中文。

我对小麦和用小麦制作的食物有过敏反应。

如果我吃了含小麦以及加防腐剂的食物，即使是少量的也会导致我发病。

如果可能的话，麻烦和厨师讲一下，我吃的食物中不能含有小麦，防腐剂，稳定剂，并请选一份我能够放心享用的饭菜。

谢谢您的合作。

GLUTEN INTOLERANCE CARD

我不懂中文。

我患有腹腔病。

如果我吃了含小麦，黑麦，燕麦，荞麦，大麦，小米，黑小麦，麦芽以及任何以这些谷物为原料的食物，或含化学添加剂，稳定剂的食物，我就会生病。

我可以吃玉米和大米做的食物。

如果可能的话，麻烦和厨师讲一下，我吃的食物中不能含有小麦，防腐剂，稳定剂，并请选一份我能够放心享用的饭菜。

多谢合作。

Recipe Acknowledgments

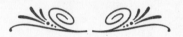

Cold Sauce "Hot Stuff" Pasta and Pasta Rustica; reprinted by permission of Sheila Lukins.

Corn and Lobster Pie in a Chili-Polenta Crust; copyright © 1994 by The New York Times Company. Reprinted by permission.

Banana Financier; reprinted by permission of Alex Cormier.

Mexican Lasagne; adapted from *The Frog Commissary Cookbook*. Reprinted by permission of Ed Barranco and George Georgiou.

Pumpkin Prosciutto Gnocchi and Jeremy's Peanut Butter and Jelly Cookies; reprinted by permission of Beth Hillson.

Abiquiu Hot Corn Soufflé; reprinted by permission of John Rivera Sedlar.

Thai-jitas; reprinted by permission of Jim Burns.

All-Corn Biscotti; reprinted by permission of Nick Malgieri.

Grown-Up Macaroni and Cheese and Mmmmmmmmmacaroni and Cheese; reprinted by permission of Caroline Winge-Bogar.

Risotto Primavera; reprinted by permission of Angelo Peloni.

Queen Mother Cake; reprinted by permission of Lynn Jamison.

Cornmeal Porridge with Dried Fruit; courtesy *Gourmet*. Copyright © 1991 by Conde Nast Publications, Inc.

Wheat-Free Brownies; reprinted by permission of Barbara Burns.

Yeast-Rising Thick Pizza Crust; reprinted by permission of Henry Holt and Company.

"Authentic" Happy Birthday Cake and "Authentic Sour Cream Ganache"; reprinted by permission of Steven Rice.

Index

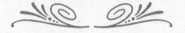

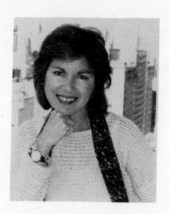

About the Author

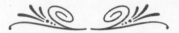

Jax Peters Lowell spent the first twenty years of her working life as an advertising writer and creative director, making do with rice cakes and carrot sticks while her colleagues gorged on prune Danish and pizza during crises, commercial shoots, brainstorming sessions, and other protracted periods of stress. Despite such deprivation, *Advertising Age* named Lowell one of the industry's "Best and Brightest Women" in 1988.

Lowell made her debut as a full-time author in 1995 with her first novel, *Mothers*, which is soon to be a major motion picture, and this, her first work of nonfiction. She is currently hard at work on a second novel.

A native New Yorker who now lives in Philadelphia with her husband, John, two cats, several cartons of rice pasta, and a bread machine, Lowell was diagnosed with celiac disease in 1981.